Sharon Telle
Judith V. Sa
Editors

The Transition
from Welfare to Work:
Processes, Challenges,
and Outcomes

The Transition from Welfare to Work: Processes, Challenges, and Outcomes has been co-published simultaneously as *Journal of Prevention & Intervention in the Community*, Volume 23, Numbers 1/2 2002.

Pre-publication
REVIEWS,
COMMENTARIES,
EVALUATIONS . . .

"Looks beyond the political al-chemy that created the 1996 Personal Responsibility and Work Opportunity Reconciliation Act and America's 'welfare reform' system. . . . Underscores that there are no quick fixes to poverty."

Philip Nyden, PhD
Professor of Sociology and Director, Center for Urban Research and Learning, Loyola University of Chicago

S

The Transition
from Welfare to Work:
Processes, Challenges,
and Outcomes

The Transition from Welfare to Work: Processes, Challenges, and Outcomes has been co-published simultaneously as *Journal of Prevention & Intervention in the Community*, Volume 23, Numbers 1/2 2002.

The *Journal of Prevention & Intervention in the Community*™ Monographic "Separates" (formerly the *Prevention in Human Services* series)*

For information on previous issues of *Prevention in Human Services,* edited by Robert E. Hess, please contact: The Haworth Press, Inc., 10 Alice Street, Binghamton, NY 13904-1580 USA.

Below is a list of "separates," which in serials librarianship means a special issue simultaneously published as a special journal issue or double-issue *and* as a "separate" hardbound monograph. (This is a format which we also call a "DocuSerial.")

"Separates" are published because specialized libraries or professionals may wish to purchase a specific thematic issue by itself in a format which can be separately cataloged and shelved, as opposed to purchasing the journal on an on-going basis. Faculty members may also more easily consider a "separate" for classroom adoption.

"Separates" are carefully classified separately with the major book jobbers so that the journal tie-in can be noted on new book order slips to avoid duplicate purchasing.

You may wish to visit Haworth's website at . . .

http://www.HaworthPress.com

. . . to search our online catalog for complete tables of contents of these separates and related publications.

You may also call 1-800-HAWORTH (outside US/Canada: 607-722-5857), or Fax 1-800-895-0582 (outside US/Canada: 607-771-0012), or e-mail at:

getinfo@haworthpressinc.com

The Transition from Welfare to Work: Processes, Challenges, and Outcomes, edited by Sharon Telleen, PhD, and Judith V. Sayad (Vol. 23, No. 1/2, 2002). *A comprehensive examination of the welfare-to-work initiatives surrounding the major reform of United States welfare legislation in 1996.*

Prevention Issues for Women's Health in the New Millennium, edited by Wendee M. Wechsberg, PhD (Vol. 22, No. 2, 2001). *"Helpful to service providers as well as researchers . . . A USEFUL ANCILLARY TEXTBOOK for courses addressing women's health issues. Covers a wide range of health issues affecting women." (Sherry Deren, PhD, Director, Center for Drug Use and HIV Research, National Drug Research Institute, New York City)*

Workplace Safety: Individual Differences in Behavior, edited by Alice F. Stuhlmacher, PhD, and Douglas F. Cellar, PhD (Vol. 22, No. 1, 2001). Workplace Safety: Individual Differences in Behavior *examines safety behavior and outlines practical interventions to help increase safety awareness. Individual differences are relevant to a variety of settings including the workplace, public spaces, and motor vehicles. This book takes a look at ways of defining and measuring safety as well as a variety of individual differences like gender, job knowledge, conscientiousness, self-efficacy, risk avoidance, and stress tolerance that are important in creating safety interventions and improving the selection and training of employees.* Workplace Safety *takes an incisive look at these issues with a unique focus on the way individual differences in people impact safety behavior in the real world.*

People with Disabilities: Empowerment and Community Action, edited by Christopher B. Keys, PhD, and Peter W. Dowrick, PhD (Vol. 21, No. 2, 2001). *"Timely and useful . . . provides valuable lessons and guidance for everyone involved in the disability movement. This book is a must-read for researchers and practitioners interested in disability rights issues!" (Karen M. Ward, EdD, Director, Center for Human Development; Associate Professor, University of Alaska, Anchorage)*

Family Systems/Family Therapy: Applications for Clinical Practice, edited by Joan D. Atwood, PhD (Vol. 21, No. 1, 2001). *Examines family therapy issues in the context of the larger systems of health, law, and education and suggests ways family therapists can effectively use an intersystems approach.*

HIV/AIDS Prevention: Current Issues in Community Practice, edited by Doreen D. Salina, PhD (Vol. 19, No. 1, 2000). *Helps researchers and psychologists explore specific methods of improving HIV/AIDS prevention research.*

Educating Students to Make-a-Difference: Community-Based Service Learning, edited by Joseph R. Ferrari, PhD, and Judith G. Chapman, PhD (Vol. 18, No. 1/2, 1999). *"There is something here for everyone interested in the social psychology of service-learning." (Frank Bernt, PhD, Associate Professor, St. Joseph's University)*

Program Implementation in Preventive Trials, edited by Joseph A. Durlak and Joseph R. Ferrari, PhD (Vol. 17, No. 2, 1998). *"Fills an important gap in preventive research. . . . Highlights an array of important questions related to implementation and demonstrates just how good community-based intervention programs can be when issues related to implementation are taken seriously." (Judy Primavera, PhD, Associate Professor of Psychology, Fairfield University, Fairfield, Connecticut)*

Preventing Drunk Driving, edited by Elsie R. Shore, PhD, and Joseph R. Ferrari, PhD (Vol. 17, No. 1, 1998). *"A must read for anyone interested in reducing the needless injuries and death caused by the drunk driver." (Terrance D. Schiavone, President, National Commission Against Drunk Driving, Washington, DC)*

Manhood Development in Urban African-American Communities, edited by Roderick J. Watts, PhD, and Robert J. Jagers (Vol. 16, No. 1/2, 1998). *"Watts and Jagers provide the much-needed foundational and baseline information and research that begins to philosophically and empirically validate the importance of understanding culture, oppression, and gender when working with males in urban African-American communities." (Paul Hill, Jr., MSW, LISW, ACSW, East End Neighborhood House, Cleveland, Ohio)*

Diversity Within the Homeless Population: Implications for Intervention, edited by Elizabeth M. Smith, PhD, and Joseph R. Ferrari, PhD (Vol. 15, No. 2, 1997). *"Examines why homelessness is increasing, as well as treatment options, case management techniques, and community intervention programs that can be used to prevent homelessness." (American Public Welfare Association)*

Education in Community Psychology: Models for Graduate and Undergraduate Programs, edited by Clifford R. O'Donnell, PhD, and Joseph R. Ferrari, PhD (Vol. 15, No. 1, 1997). *"An invaluable resource for students seeking graduate training in community psychology . . . [and will] also serve faculty who want to improve undergraduate teaching and graduate programs." (Marybeth Shinn, PhD, Professor of Psychology and Coordinator, Community Doctoral Program, New York University, New York, New York)*

Adolescent Health Care: Program Designs and Services, edited by John S. Wodarski, PhD, Marvin D. Feit, PhD, and Joseph R. Ferrari, PhD (Vol. 14, No. 1/2, 1997). *Devoted to helping practitioners address the problems of our adolescents through the use of preventive interventions based on sound empirical data.*

Preventing Illness Among People with Coronary Heart Disease, edited by John D. Piette, PhD, Robert M. Kaplan, PhD, and Joseph R. Ferrari, PhD (Vol. 13, No. 1/2, 1996). *"A useful contribution to the interaction of physical health, mental health, and the behavioral interventions for patients with CHD." (Public Health: The Journal of the Society of Public Health)*

Sexual Assault and Abuse: Sociocultural Context of Prevention, edited by Carolyn F. Swift, PhD* (Vol. 12, No. 2, 1995). *"Delivers a cornucopia for all who are concerned with the primary prevention of these damaging and degrading acts." (George J. McCall, PhD, Professor of Sociology and Public Administration, University of Missouri)*

International Approaches to Prevention in Mental Health and Human Services, edited by Robert E. Hess, PhD, and Wolfgang Stark* (Vol. 12, No. 1, 1995). *Increases knowledge of prevention strategies from around the world.*

Self-Help and Mutual Aid Groups: International and Multicultural Perspectives, edited by Francine Lavoie, PhD, Thomasina Borkman, PhD, and Benjamin Gidron* (Vol. 11, No. 1/2, 1995). *"A helpful orientation and overview, as well as useful data and methodological suggestions." (International Journal of Group Psychotherapy)*

Prevention and School Transitions, edited by Leonard A. Jason, PhD, Karen E. Danner, and Karen S. Kurasaki, MA* (Vol. 10, No. 2, 1994). *"A collection of studies by leading ecological and systems-oriented theorists in the area of school transitions, describing the stressors, personal resources available, and coping strategies among different groups of children and adolescents undergoing school transitions." (Reference & Research Book News)*

Religion and Prevention in Mental Health: Research, Vision, and Action, edited by Kenneth I. Pargament, PhD, Kenneth I. Maton, PhD, and Robert E. Hess, PhD* (Vol. 9, No. 2 & Vol. 10, No. 1, 1992). *"The authors provide an admirable framework for considering the important, yet often overlooked, differences in theological perspectives." (Family Relations)*

Families as Nurturing Systems: Support Across the Life Span, edited by Donald G. Unger, PhD, and Douglas R. Powell, PhD* (Vol. 9, No. 1, 1991). *"A useful book for anyone thinking about alternative ways of delivering a mental health service." (British Journal of Psychiatry)*

Ethical Implications of Primary Prevention, edited by Gloria B. Levin, PhD, and Edison J. Trickett, PhD* (Vol. 8, No. 2, 1991). *"A thoughtful and thought-provoking summary of ethical issues related to intervention programs and community research." (Betty Tableman, MPA, Director, Division of Prevention Services and Demonstration Projects, Michigan Department of Mental Health, Lansing). Here is the first systematic and focused treatment of the ethical implications of primary prevention practice and research.*

Career Stress in Changing Times, edited by James Campbell Quick, PhD, MBA, Robert E. Hess, PhD, Jared Hermalin, PhD, and Jonathan D. Quick, MD* (Vol. 8, No. 1, 1990). *"A well-organized book. . . . It deals with planning a career and career changes and the stresses involved." (American Association of Psychiatric Administrators)*

Prevention in Community Mental Health Centers, edited by Robert E. Hess, PhD, and John Morgan, PhD* (Vol. 7, No. 2, 1990). *"A fascinating bird's-eye view of six significant programs of preventive care which have survived the rise and fall of preventive psychiatry in the U.S." (British Journal of Psychiatry)*

Protecting the Children: Strategies for Optimizing Emotional and Behavioral Development, edited by Raymond P. Lorion, PhD* (Vol. 7, No. 1, 1990). *"This is a masterfully conceptualized and edited volume presenting theory-driven, empirically based, developmentally oriented prevention." (Michael C. Roberts, PhD, Professor of Psychology, The University of Alabama)*

The National Mental Health Association: Eighty Years of Involvement in the Field of Prevention, edited by Robert E. Hess, PhD, and Jean DeLeon, PhD* (Vol. 6, No. 2, 1989). *"As a family life educator interested in both the history of the field, current efforts, and especially the evaluation of programs, I find this book quite interesting. I enjoyed reviewing it and believe that I will return to it many times. It is also a book I will recommend to students." (Family Relations)*

A Guide to Conducting Prevention Research in the Community: First Steps, by James G. Kelly, PhD, Nancy Dassoff, PhD, Ira Levin, PhD, Janice Schreckengost, MA, AB, Stephen P. Stelzner, PhD, and B. Eileen Altman, PhD* (Vol. 6, No. 1, 1989). *"An invaluable compendium for the prevention practitioner, as well as the researcher, laying out the essentials for developing effective prevention programs in the community. . . . This is a book which should be in the prevention practitioner's library, to read, re-read, and ponder." (The Community Psychologist)*

Prevention: Toward a Multidisciplinary Approach, edited by Leonard A. Jason, PhD, Robert D. Felner, PhD, John N. Moritsugu, PhD, and Robert E. Hess, PhD* (Vol. 5, No. 2, 1987). *"Will not only be of intellectual value to the professional but also to students in courses aimed at presenting a refreshingly comprehensive picture of the conceptual and practical relationships between community and prevention." (Seymour B. Sarason, Associate Professor of Psychology, Yale University)*

Prevention and Health: Directions for Policy and Practice, edited by Alfred H. Katz, PhD, Jared A. Hermalin, PhD, and Robert E. Hess, PhD* (Vol. 5, No. 1, 1987). *Read about the most current efforts being undertaken to promote better health.*

The Ecology of Prevention: Illustrating Mental Health Consultation, edited by James G. Kelly, PhD, and Robert E. Hess, PhD* (Vol. 4, No. 3/4, 1987). *"Will provide the consultant with a very useful framework and the student with an appreciation for the time and commitment necessary to bring about lasting changes of a preventive nature." (The Community Psychologist)*

Beyond the Individual: Environmental Approaches and Prevention, edited by Abraham Wandersman, PhD, and Robert E. Hess, PhD* (Vol. 4, No. 1/2, 1985). *"This excellent book has immediate appeal for those involved with environmental psychology . . . likely to be of great interest to those working in the areas of community psychology, planning, and design." (Australian Journal of Psychology)*

Prevention: The Michigan Experience, edited by Betty Tableman, MPA, and Robert E. Hess, PhD* (Vol. 3, No. 4, 1985). *An in-depth look at one state's outstanding prevention programs.*

Studies in Empowerment: Steps Toward Understanding and Action, edited by Julian Rappaport, Carolyn Swift, and Robert E. Hess, PhD* (Vol. 3, No. 2/3, 1984). *"Provides diverse applications of the empowerment model to the promotion of mental health and the prevention of mental illness." (Prevention Forum Newsline)*

Aging and Prevention: New Approaches for Preventing Health and Mental Health Problems in Older Adults, edited by Sharon P. Simson, Laura Wilson, Jared Hermalin, PhD, and Robert E. Hess, PhD* (Vol. 3, No. 1, 1983). *"Highly recommended for professionals and laymen interested in modern viewpoints and techniques for avoiding many physical and mental health problems of the elderly. Written by highly qualified contributors with extensive experience in their respective fields." (The Clinical Gerontologist)*

Strategies for Needs Assessment in Prevention, edited by Alex Zautra, Kenneth Bachrach, and Robert E. Hess, PhD* (Vol. 2, No. 4, 1983). *"An excellent survey on applied techniques for doing needs assessments. . . . It should be on the shelf of anyone involved in prevention." (Journal of Pediatric Psychology)*

Innovations in Prevention, edited by Robert E. Hess, PhD, and Jared Hermalin, PhD* (Vol. 2, No. 3, 1983). *An exciting book that provides invaluable insights on effective prevention programs.*

Rx Television: Enhancing the Preventive Impact of TV, edited by Joyce Sprafkin, Carolyn Swift, PhD, and Robert E. Hess, PhD* (Vol. 2, No. 1/2, 1983). *"The successful interventions reported in this volume make interesting reading on two grounds. First, they show quite clearly how powerful television can be in molding children. Second, they illustrate how this power can be used for good ends." (Contemporary Psychology)*

Early Intervention Programs for Infants, edited by Howard A. Moss, MD, Robert E. Hess, PhD, and Carolyn Swift, PhD* (Vol. 1, No. 4, 1982). *"A useful resource book for those child psychiatrists, paediatricians, and psychologists interested in early intervention and prevention." (The Royal College of Psychiatrists)*

Helping People to Help Themselves: Self-Help and Prevention, edited by Leonard D. Borman, PhD, Leslie E. Borck, PhD, Robert E. Hess, PhD, and Frank L. Pasquale* (Vol. 1, No. 3, 1982). *"A timely volume . . . a mine of information for interested clinicians, and should stimulate those wishing to do systematic research in the self-help area." (The Journal of Nervous and Mental Disease)*

Evaluation and Prevention in Human Services, edited by Jared Hermalin, PhD, and Jonathan A. Morell, PhD* (Vol. 1, No. 1/2, 1982). *Features methods and problems related to the evaluation of prevention programs.*

The Transition from Welfare to Work: Processes, Challenges, and Outcomes has been co-published simultaneously as *Journal of Prevention & Intervention in the Community*™, Volume 23, Numbers 1/2 2002.

The Haworth Press, Inc., 10 Alice Street, Binghamton, NY 13904-1580 USA

Cover design by Thomas J. Mayshock Jr.

Library of Congress Cataloging-in-Publication Data

The transition from welfare to work : processes, challenges, and outcomes / Sharon Telleen, Judith V. Sayad, editors.
     p. cm.
Co-published simultaneously as Journal of Prevention & Intervention in the Community, Volume 23, Numbers 1/2 2002.
Includes bibliographical references and index.
     ISBN 0-7890-1942-6 (hard : alk. paper) – ISBN 0-7890-1943-4 (pbk : alk. paper)
1. Public welfare–United States. 2. Welfare recipients–Employment–United States. I. Telleen, Sharon. II. Sayad, Judith V.
HV95 .T673 2002
361.6′8′0973–dc21

2002010969

The Transition
from Welfare to Work:
Processes, Challenges,
and Outcomes

Sharon Telleen, PhD
Judith V. Sayad
Editors

The Transition from Welfare to Work: Processes, Challenges, and Outcomes has been co-published simultaneously as *Journal of Prevention & Intervention in the Community*, Volume 23, Numbers 1/2 2002.

The Haworth Press, Inc.
New York • London • Oxford

Indexing, Abstracting & Website/Internet Coverage

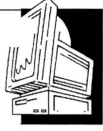

This section provides you with a list of major indexing & abstracting services. That is to say, each service began covering this periodical during the year noted in the right column. Most Websites which are listed below have indicated that they will either post, disseminate, compile, archive, cite or alert their own Website users with research-based content from this work. (This list is as current as the copyright date of this publication.)

(continued)

(continued)

*Special Bibliographic Notes related to special journal issues
(separates) and indexing/abstracting:*

- indexing/abstracting services in this list will also cover material in any "separate" that is co-published simultaneously with Haworth's special thematic journal issue or DocuSerial. Indexing/abstracting usually covers material at the article/chapter level.
- monographic co-editions are intended for either non-subscribers or libraries which intend to purchase a second copy for their circulating collections.
- monographic co-editions are reported to all jobbers/wholesalers/approval plans. The source journal is listed as the "series" to assist the prevention of duplicate purchasing in the same manner utilized for books-in-series.
- to facilitate user/access services all indexing/abstracting services are encouraged to utilize the co-indexing entry note indicated at the bottom of the first page of each article/chapter/contribution.
- this is intended to assist a library user of any reference tool (whether print, electronic, online, or CD-ROM) to locate the monographic version if the library has purchased this version but not a subscription to the source journal.
- individual articles/chapters in any Haworth publication are also available through the Haworth Document Delivery Service (HDDS).

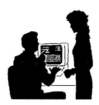

The Transition from Welfare to Work: Processes, Challenges, and Outcomes

CONTENTS

ABOUT THE EDITORS

Sharon Telleen, PhD, is Visiting Research Associate Professor in the Department of Sociology at the University of Illinois at Chicago. Dr. Telleen's areas of specialization include child development, community psychology, and maternal and child health. She has been the principal investigator of federal research grants studying the effect of social support on use of child health services by low-income immigrant Latino families, the impact of welfare, income and neighborhood characteristics on child health outcomes, and the effectiveness of case management for women receiving Medicaid.

Judith V. Sayad is a project coordinator in the Department of Sociology and the School of Public Health, University of Illinois at Chicago. Sayad has spent most of her career as an occupational health and safety professional serving small manufacturers. She also worked for The Center for Neighborhood Technology in Chicago, where she covered the environmental beat for *The Neighborhood Works*. She has served as managing editor for a number of publications on community research.

The editors gratefully acknowledge the colleagues who made it possible for us to produce this volume. Dr. Edward Mensah, health economist at UIC's School of Public Health, provided invaluable assistance concerning the economics of welfare reform and helped us and Laura Connolly to present a detailed and accessible discussion of these complex issues. We also thank Dr. William R. Kelley whose acumen as a social scientist and attention to detail is directly responsible for the completion of this project.

Challenges of Welfare Reform

Sharon Telleen

University of Illinois at Chicago

We are entering a period of time in which it will be necessary to examine the success of the current welfare law, rules and regulations. The 1996 Personal Responsibility and Work Opportunity Reconciliation Act brought a fundamental change in the structure of the provision of support to needy families. (In this volume Banias provides a description of these changes.) The major new program created by the Act, Temporary Assistance to Needy Families (TANF), must be reauthorized in 2002; with this comes the need for a broad assessment of the progress of these welfare programs.

In reexamining the law it is important to look at the impact of the law's major provisions in light of its intents and goals. Among the purposes of the law was to help former welfare recipients become self-sufficient by obtaining jobs, retaining jobs and increasing their earnings and incomes through work. These were not the only goals of the legislation, however. An increase in participation in the labor force was intended to serve other social goals, as well. To accomplish the former was also intended to have the effect, among others, of reducing welfare case loads, increasing the number of former welfare recipients in the workforce, and reducing the number of families and children living in poverty.

Address correspondence to: Sharon Telleen, Department of Sociology, University of Illinois at Chicago, 1007 W. Harrison Street, M/C 312, Chicago, IL 60607.

[Haworth co-indexing entry note]: "Challenges of Welfare Reform." Telleen, Sharon. Co-published simultaneously in *Journal of Prevention & Intervention in the Community* (The Haworth Press, Inc.) Vol. 23, No. 1/2, 2002, pp. 1- 5; and: *The Transition from Welfare to Work: Processes, Challenges, and Outcomes* (ed: Sharon Telleen, and Judith V. Sayad) The Haworth Press, Inc., 2002, pp. 1- 5. Single or multiple copies of this article are available for a fee from The Haworth Document Delivery Service [1-800-HAWORTH, 9:00 a.m. - 5:00 p.m. (EST). E-mail address: getinfo@haworthpressinc.com].

Aggregate indicators suggest that the first set of goals has, at least to some extent, been achieved. Welfare caseloads have declined. Work among single mothers has increased. In 1999 the rate of child poverty was 16.3%, down from a high of 22% in 1993 (Falk et al., 2001).

Aggregate indicators do not, however, reveal much about the transition from welfare to work as a process, and it is the process that determines whether the welfare reforms have been effective. If women leave the case-loads without adequate preparation for a lifetime of work, rather than be-cause they found a job, then the welfare caseload may be a misleading indicator. If women leave welfare only to discover that they are now part of the uninsured working poor, then the rate of women at work may not be a good indicator of the well-being of their families. Only an understanding of the internal structure of the process, then, will reveal if the welfare-to-work process was effective. If it was not, then superficial improvement in "the numbers" may conceal intrinsic flaws that could have negative conse-quences later. This volume addresses the problem of understanding the hu-man processes involved in the transition from welfare to work, along with what is known about its impact on the families involved and the likely ulti-mate outcomes of the shift from cash assistance to a work-first approach.

THE PROCESS OF ORIENTING A LIFE TOWARDS WORK

The demand that mothers on welfare enter the workforce requires these women to restructure their lives in such a way that they are able to take jobs. Every other aspect of a woman's life must take a form that will enable her to go to work. For that reason all other aspects of her life be-come relevant to understanding her ability to make the transition from welfare to work. The authors of three papers in this volume address this question. Telleen and Andes study barriers to work that were identified by case managers in a program that offered intensive individual support to women trying to make the transition to work. They discovered that the context within which women live has a profound effect on the wel-fare-to-work transition. Looking at a smaller social unit, Crittenden and her colleagues focus on how a mother's transition to work is affected by her place in her and her family's life cycle, particularly the timing of the birth of children, their early and later preschool years, and their early years in elementary school. Hair and her colleagues turn to more individ-ual qualities, such as maternal depression and literacy, to tease out the dif-fering impacts of the two on both maternal success in employment and two important outcomes for their children.

OUTCOMES

What, then, are the outcomes for women participating in welfare-to-work programs? In two articles, Ferrari and his colleagues examine whether participation in job training in itself has an effect on perceived self-efficacy among welfare recipients.

Once women have moved from welfare to work, what is known about the impact of this transition on the health and well-being of the women and their families? For example, are women who are eligible for transitional Medicaid receiving services? Rojas Smith and her colleagues examine the extent to which information is being collected that would help answer questions such as this.

Finally, what data do we have to demonstrate whether impoverished families are doing better under the welfare-to-work provisions of TANF than under the previous program of AFDC? By making use of a nearly unique conjunction of historical legislative circumstances, Connolly has been able to compare the earnings and incomes of low-income women under the former AFDC program with those of women participating in work-first programs, and suggests that their total incomes may not be significantly better. Connolly uses the Current Population Survey to construct a synthetic panel that estimates year-to-year changes and the way they are affected by different conditions. Because Connolly's research was conducted prior to the 1996 legislation, she was able to compare the traditional welfare cash assistance program (which served as a control group) to state-level welfare waiver programs, which included work-first and work-requirement experimental groups. Her ability to compare control and experimental groups provides valuable information. The experimental (state waiver) groups became the basis for the 1996 welfare legislation; when the new legislation created uniformity among the state programs a control group was no longer possible.

Even if incomes may not have grown any more rapidly than they would have without welfare reform, have those who left welfare nevertheless also left poverty? Quite possibly not. Though welfare recipients are finding jobs, their wages and total household income are not enough to lift them out of poverty. Most former welfare recipients are being paid the minimum wage or just slightly higher, which is not enough to make them totally self-sufficient. On the minimum wage it is extremely difficult to support children and find housing, food and clothing for a family.

Among the hardest hit are the urban poor. Wages in both rural and urban areas are just above the minimum wage, but as Connolly points out, the growth of earnings and household income among the poor are even less in urban areas than in rural areas.

What must be done to help the urban poor do better? At this point the other studies in the volume may prove to be useful a second time. The article by Rojas Smith suggests, first, that policy analysts continue to need more and better information on how people are doing. The articles by Crittenden et al., Hair et al., and Telleen and Andes each identify personal, familial, or larger community forces at play in the lives of welfare recipients. These forces, which so often act as barriers to employment, could be neutralized or converted into assets with appropriate programs to address them.

The emphasis in the current law on obtaining work first, with limited weeks in job skills training counting toward the work requirement, makes programs of instruction even more important for the success of welfare-to-work initiatives. Job search strategies may need to be taught. Socialization to a job and workplace becomes key for first-time job seekers. Corporations, such as Marriott, have played a vital role in acclimating former welfare recipients to the workplace and in providing job skills training. The results of the various forms of instruction have taken or increased importance in the current economic downturn.

The role of functional literacy on job search strategy and employment will need to be addressed. More generally, it is important to understand and accept the extent of investment in human capital that will be necessary for a large number of individuals to leave welfare and obtain the type of job that could enable economic self-sufficiency.

Finally, one thing that does appear to help lift low-income women and children out of poverty is the financial contribution of the father, a second parent. For those circumstances in which the father is absent, the Child Support Enforcement program of the 1996 legislation increased the level of child support that could be demanded from fathers for their children. More than money, though, it seems to be the case that when both parents are present, it is not only the combined wages of both parents but the addition of the social capital which the second parent brings to the family that helps to keep the family running. It may be useful to consider policies that serve to help keep families together under conditions of stress.

All of this is based on the presumption that the goal of welfare reform was to help raise families to a level of self-sufficiency, to make it possible for welfare recipients and their children to provide themselves greater access to resources of various kinds than was possible under the old program. This has not addressed arguments that would suggest that welfare reform is good in itself, regardless of its impact on the health and well-being of adults and their children. Whether someone is part of the working poor or a parent raising children with public cash assistance, to substitute one form of poverty for another would be no reform. Future research, including longitudinal studies of TANF recipients, is important in monitoring the factors that contribute to positive employment, family outcomes, and the impact on children.

REFERENCE

Falk, G., Burke, V., Gish, M., Solomon-Fears, C., Richardson, J., Spar, K. (2001). Welfare reform reauthorization: brief summary of issues for the 107th Congress. Washington, DC: Library of Congress, Congressional Research Service Report RS 20766.

The Effects of Welfare-to-Work Legislation on Children and Mothers: A Legal Overview

Irene Banias

College of Law, DePaul University

SUMMARY. Current welfare reform efforts are based upon the challenges brought since the August 1996 passage of the Personal Responsibility and Work Opportunity Reconciliation Act (P.L. 104-193), which eliminated individual and family entitlement to assistance and ended one of the nation's safety nets for poor families, the 60-year-old program, Aid to Families with Dependent Children (AFDC). This new law provides states with block grants and creates financial incentives for states to run mandatory, work-focused welfare-to-work programs. An overview of the law is presented including participation standards, work requirements, time limits, enforcement strategies, and program exemptions. Funding mechanisms and other program mechanics are discussed. *[Article copies available for a fee from The Haworth Document Delivery Service: 1-800-HAWORTH. E-mail address: <getinfo@haworthpressinc. com> Website: <http://www.HaworthPress.com> © 2002 by The Haworth Press, Inc. All rights reserved.]*

KEYWORDS. Welfare reform, program requirements, federal law

Address correspondence to: Irene Banias, Fulbright Scholar, University of Bosophorus, Istanbul, Turkey (E-mail: ibanias@yahoo.com).

[Haworth co-indexing entry note]: "The Effects of Welfare-to-Work Legislation on Children and Mothers: A Legal Overview." Banias, Irene. Co-published simultaneously in *Journal of Prevention & Intervention in the Community* (The Haworth Press, Inc.) Vol. 23, No. 1/2, 2002, pp. 7-12; and: *The Transition from Welfare to Work: Processes, Challenges, and Outcomes* (ed: Sharon Telleen, and Judith V. Sayad) The Haworth Press, Inc., 2002, pp. 7-12. Single or multiple copies of this article are available for a fee from The Haworth Document Delivery Service [1-800-HAWORTH, 9:00 a.m. - 5:00 p.m. (EST). E-mail address: getinfo@haworthpressinc.com].

In August 1996, Congress passed the Personal Responsibility and Work Opportunity Reconciliation Act (P.L. 104-193), which eliminated individual and family entitlement to assistance and ended one of the nation's safety nets for poor families, the 60-year-old program, Aid to Families with Dependent Children (AFDC). Temporary Assistance for Needy Families (TANF), which replaced AFDC, Emergency Assistance (EA) and Job Opportunities and Basic Skills Training (JOBS), is a funding mechanism that provides states with block grants and creates financial incentives for states to run mandatory, work-focused welfare-to-work programs. While these types of programs are not new, certain aspects of the 1996 law are of particular importance. Federal funds cannot be used to support most families on welfare for longer than five years, and states have the option to set shorter time limits. States face financial penalties if they fail to meet TANF-defined "participation standards," which require large proportions of welfare recipients to be working or in work-related activities. In addition, states must have a plan for how they will require recipients to work after two years of assistance.

Five years after the passage of welfare reform there has been a dramatic increase in employment of welfare recipients. Analysis of all available sources of information shows that the employment rate of current and former TANF recipients has increased significantly. The percentage of working recipients in 1999 reached 33%, compared to less than 7% in 1992 and 11% in 1996 (Health and Human Services, 2000). The majority of recipients who were working were in paid employment (85% of those working) while others were engaged in work experience and community service. Welfare caseloads have declined since welfare reform, from 5.1 million AFDC families in March 1994, to 2.2 million families in June 2000. Food stamp caseloads have also declined (Falk, G. et al., 2001).

Has the nation met the objectives of welfare reform? Not long ago ex-president Clinton, Congress and governors proclaimed success, while many advocates worried about those who have fallen through the cracks. Behind these opinions lie different standards for judging welfare. Is welfare primarily about reducing caseloads, reducing poverty or hardship, requiring work, promoting marriage, or improving the emotional and physical well-being of children (Weil, A., 2001)?

The purpose of this article is to introduce the pertinent provisions of the law.

OVERVIEW OF THE WELFARE LAW

The block grants to the states represent a consolidation of AFDC, Emergency Assistance (EA), and JOBS into a single capped entitlement to states–Temporary Assistance to Needy Families (TANF). The states were required to implement their block grants programs by July 1, 1997, subject to review for completeness by the Department of Health and Human Services.

Funding

The funding allocated for the total cash assistance block grant is approximately $16.4 billion for each year from fiscal year 1996 to fiscal year 2002. The fixed amount that each state receives is based on its previous expenditures on AFDC, EA and JOBS, equal to or greater of: (1) 1/3 of the total of federal payments for these programs in fiscal years 1992-1994; (2) federal payments in fiscal year 1994, plus additional EA funding for some states; or (3) estimated federal payments in fiscal year 1995.

Time Limits for Cash Assistance

Under the new welfare law, families who have received federally funded assistance for five cumulative years (or less at state option) will be ineligible for additional cash aid. States are permitted to exempt up to 20% of their caseload from the time limit, and states have the option to provide non-cash assistance and vouchers to families that reach the federal time limit using Social Services Block Grant or state funds.

Work Requirements

With only a few exceptions, under the new law recipients must work after two years on assistance. Twenty-five percent of all families in each state should be engaged in work activities or have left the rolls in fiscal year 1997, rising to 50% in fiscal year 2002 (states were to have been penalized for not reaching these rates). The rate for two-parent families increased from 75% to 90% by fiscal year 1999.

Single-parent recipients are required to work 20 hours per week, increasing to at least 30 hours per week by fiscal year 2000. Single parents with a child under age six may meet the requirement by working 20 hours per week. Two-parent families must work 35 hours per week.

Exemptions. There are two classes of exemptions: (a) Single parents of children under age six who cannot find child care will not be penalized for failure to meet work requirements. States can also exempt single parents with children under age 1 and disregard these individuals in the calculation of participation rates for up to 12 months. (b) For two-parent families, the second spouse is required to participate 20 hours per week in work activities if they receive federally funded child care (and are not disabled or caring for a disabled child). Individuals who receive assistance for two months and are not working or exempt from the work requirements are required to participate in community service, with the hours and tasks to be determined by the state (states can opt-out of this provision).

Work Activities

Activities that count toward state work requirements include participation in unsubsidized or subsidized employment, on-the-job training, work experience, community service, 12 months of vocational training, or providing child care services to individuals who are participating in community service. Up to six weeks of job search (no more than four consecutive weeks) would count toward the work requirement. There is a limit; no more than 20% of each state's caseload may count toward the work requirement solely by participating in vocational training or being a teen parent in secondary school.

Personal Employability Plans

Under the new plan, states are required to make an initial assessment of recipients' skills. States have the option of developing personal responsibility plans for recipients, identifying the education, training, and job placement services needed to move into the workforce.

Penalties

Failure to comply with federal requirements exposes states to penalties including the following: (a) a penalty of 5% is imposed on a state's block grant for failure to meet the work participation rate in the first year increasing by 2% per year for each consecutive failure (with a cap of 21%); (b) a reduction of 4% for failure to submit required reports; (c) a reduction of up to 2% for failure to participate in the Income and Eligibility

Verification System; (d) for misuse of funds, the amount equal to the funds misused with an additional 5% penalty if the misuse was intentional; (e) up to 5% penalty for failing to comply with the five-year limit on federally funded assistance; and (f) a 5% penalty for failing to maintain assistance to a parent who cannot obtain child care for a child under age 6.

State Maintenance of Effort Requirements

States are required to maintain their own spending on welfare at least 80% of fiscal year 1994 levels. States must also maintain spending at 100% of fiscal 1994 levels to access a $2 billion contingency fund designed to assist states affected by high population growth or economic downturn. In addition, states must maintain 100% of fiscal years 1994 or 1995 spending on child care (whichever is greater) to access additional child care funds beyond their initial allotment.

Performance Bonus to Reward Work

One billion dollars as a performance bonus will be available between fiscal years 1999 and 2003 to reward states for moving welfare recipients into jobs.

Teen Parent Provisions

Live at home and stay in school requirements. In order to receive assistance unmarried minor parents are required to live with a responsible adult or in an adult-supervised setting and participate in educational and training activities. States will be responsible for locating or assisting in locating adult-supervised settings for teens.

Teen pregnancy prevention. Starting in fiscal year 1998, $50 million per year in mandatory funds is added to appropriations of the Maternal and Child Health (MCH) Block Grant for abstinence education with the option of targeting the funds to high-risk groups (i.e., groups most likely to bear children out-of-wedlock).

Child Care

There is a separate allocation specifically for child care. The law authorized $13.9 billion in mandatory funding for fiscal years 1997-2002.

States receive approximately $1.2 billion of the mandatory funds each year. The remainder is available subject to state match. The law provides no child care guarantee, but single parents with children under age 6 who cannot find child care may not be penalized for failure to engage in work activities.

REFERENCES

Falk, G. et al. (2001). *Welfare Reform Reauthorization: Brief Summary of Issues for the 107th Congress*, January 4, 2001. CRS report to Congress.

United States Department of HHS, Administration for Children and Families (2000). *Third Annual Report to Congress*, p. 1.

Weil, A. (2000). *Where Is Welfare Reform Heading? San Francisco Chronicle*, September 22, 2000.

The Social Ecology
of the Transition to Work

Sharon Telleen
Steven Andes

University of Illinois at Chicago

SUMMARY. The State of Illinois provided intensive case management to assist women making the transition from welfare to work. Case managers involved in this process discovered that a variety of challenges faced the women. A social ecological approach to organizing these challenges found six distinct considerations: (1) awareness of the requirements of the law; (2) the environmental context and social norms common in a neighborhood; (3) family support, family structure and family expectations; (4) emotional well-being; (5) literacy and education; and (6) appropriate expectations of the work environment. *[Article copies available for a fee from The Haworth Document Delivery Service: 1-800-HAWORTH. E-mail address: <getinfo@haworthpressinc.com> Website: <http://www.HaworthPress.com> © 2002 by The Haworth Press, Inc. All rights reserved.]*

KEYWORDS. Low-income women, social ecology, intensive case management, TANF

Address correspondence to: Sharon Telleen, Department of Sociology, University of Illinois at Chicago, 1007 W. Harrison Street, M/C 312, Chicago, IL 60607.

[Haworth co-indexing entry note]: "The Social Ecology of the Transition to Work." Telleen, Sharon, and Steven Andes. Co-published simultaneously in *Journal of Prevention & Intervention in the Community* (The Haworth Press, Inc.) Vol. 23, No. 1/2, 2002, pp.13-39; and: *The Transition from Welfare to Work: Processes, Challenges, and Outcomes* (ed: Sharon Telleen, and Judith V. Sayad) The Haworth Press, Inc., 2002, pp.13-39. Single or multiple copies of this article are available for a fee from The Haworth Document Delivery Service [1-800-HAWORTH, 9:00 a.m. - 5:00 p.m. (EST). E-mail address: getinfo@haworthpressinc.com].

INTRODUCTION

In 1996 Congress passed P.L. 104-193, the Personal Responsibility and Work Opportunity Reconciliation Act (PRWORA).[1] Among its other provisions PRWORA replaced the entitlement program known as Aid to Families with Dependent Children (AFDC) with Temporary Assistance for Needy Families (TANF). The TANF legislation provided states with block grants and new flexibility in designing welfare programs. Based on pre-TANF research on welfare-to-work strategies, an essential element of the new law was an increased emphasis on "work first," which focused on employment search strategies and the quickest possible placement. This article reports agency staff perceptions of barriers they found when trying to implement a program developed under the new law, as well as staff perceptions of their clients' transition from welfare to work.

Under the new legislation Illinois filed a state plan in July, 1997 (Illinois Department of Public Aid, 1997). One component of this plan was the Illinois Job Advantage program. In line with the national reorientation, the Illinois Job Advantage program emphasized work first, including job searches, placement, and retention.

This study examines the types of personal barriers that were faced by women with children as they participated in the Illinois Job Advantage program. The program implemented its work-first orientation through a system of intensive case management. Since the vast majority of welfare recipients are women, any program of case management activities involving welfare recipients addresses the unique challenges faced by women with children. The study also focused on the personal barriers faced by these women because personal barriers to employment have emerged as one of the major factors in predicting employment (Danziger et al., 2000). A better understanding of the personal barriers faced by women with children will go some distance towards providing a better understanding of the conditions that must be put in place to maximize the public and private benefits of welfare reform.

Intensive focus groups were used to discover agency staff perceptions of these barriers and how they tried to respond. As case management staff in the participating agencies sought to implement Illinois Job Advantage they discovered that clients might possess a variety of personal barriers that could interfere with their movement from welfare to work. Once these barriers were identified the staff also attempted to address to these barriers as best they could. Focus group interviews made it possible for the case management staff to become more aware of and better able to describe the various kinds of barriers that were found and their responses to them.

As themes emerged from the focus group responses the study used an ecological model to define these themes. The social ecological model has repeatedly been found useful in describing and relating the many influences that affect an individual's behavior (Trickett, 1984; Telleen, 1990; Kelly, Ryan, Altman, & Stelzner, 2000).

Use of an ecological model for understanding the transition to work makes it possible to describe multiple levels of influence that, taken together, affect the transition from welfare to work for mothers with children. Agency staff responsible for implementing the program found that a mother's transition was dependent upon support from all levels: (1) her awareness of the requirements of the law; (2) the environmental context and social norms common in her neighborhood; (3) family support, family structure and family expectations; individual factors such as: (4) emotional barriers, (5) literacy and education, and (6) her expectations of the work environment.

RESEARCH ON PRE-TANF EMPLOYMENT-FOCUSED STRATEGIES

For ten years prior to the passage of PRWORA a number of states conducted large-scale rigorous studies of welfare-to-work programs (Freedman et al., 2000; Martinson, 2000). The welfare-to-work strategies found in PRWORA were shaped in part by the findings of evaluations of the Job Opportunities and Basic Skills Training Program (JOBS Program). The JOBS Program, established by the Family Support Act of 1988, contained a welfare-to-work program. The Family Support Act also called for an experimental evaluation of the economic impact of JOBS programs. This large scale evaluation is known as the National Evaluation of Welfare-to-Work Strategies (NEWWS). NEWWS has provided a number of important findings concerning the conditions that tend to lead towards or away from sustained employment.

WorkFirst Compared to Pre-Employment Training

One of the most significant findings was the importance of strategies that focused on employment first. In one of the major studies funded under NEWWS, the Manpower Demonstration Research Corporation (MDRC) reviewed 20 welfare-to-work programs for their impact on employment (Michalopoulos & Schwartz, 2000). All of these programs were established prior to the passage of TANF and most were part of state programs funded under the JOBS Program of the Family Support Act of 1988.

The study by MDRC compared the outcomes of individuals assigned to control groups with the outcomes of those assigned to one of three experimental groups. At each site MDRC used a research design in which, at the time of welfare payment, individuals were randomly assigned to either (1) a control group which did not participate in welfare-to-work programs, and individuals received cash payments only under the existing AFDC rules; or (2) an experimental group which required participation in a program that involved either (a) an employment setting (work first), (b) an education or training program, or (c) some combination of the two. The experimental groups recruited participants by requiring some portion of the individuals who made up the welfare caseload to participate in a welfare-to-work program or risk losing some or all of their welfare benefits through sanctions.

In the experimental groups five sites encouraged or required nearly all individuals to look for work, seven focused on basic education, and eight used a mixture of the two approaches. The eight that combined approaches encouraged or required participants who were more job-ready to look for work but allowed others to develop their skills through education. This variation revealed the effects of the specific programs by allowing a comparison both between the two programs, employment versus education, and between the experimental versus control groups.

In the analysis, individuals in the experimental group were subdivided into a more disadvantaged subgroup and a less disadvantaged subgroup. The more disadvantaged group was defined to include those who were long-term recipients (those who had ever been on welfare for two years or more prior to random assignment to the program), those who had not graduated from high school or those who had no earnings in the year prior to random assignment to the program. A less disadvantaged group was defined as individuals with none of these indicators.

Success of the education and work programs could vary among three dimensions: (1) increased employment and earnings; (2) reduced government spending on welfare (i.e., reducing cash assistance); and (3) increased total income. The focus was on increased earnings.

Programs that required nearly all participants to look for work from the outset had larger effects on earnings for the more disadvantaged subgroups than programs that enrolled most people initially into basic education prior to employment. Over the three-year follow-up period, employment-focused programs produced four of the five largest earnings impacts for individuals who had no earnings in the year prior to random assignment, for long-term welfare recipients, and for the more disadvantaged group overall.

Another study by MDRC showed similar results. The evaluation of the Los Angeles Job-First GAIN Program found that it raised two-year earnings and reduced welfare payments for recipients who lacked education credentials, job skills or work experience. The outcomes of the GAIN program also demonstrated that employment-focused programs can work for each of these subgroups (Freedman et al., 2000).

Barriers to Obtaining and Sustaining Employment

As part of NEWWS, MDRC also conducted an evaluation funded by the U. S. Department of Health and Human Services. This evaluation examined the effectiveness of 11 mandatory welfare-to-work programs operated in seven locales (Martinson, 2000). The study looked at the characteristics of those who were most effective in obtaining a job and remaining in the work force. Two dimensions, those of education and personal concerns, emerged as the most salient barriers to employment.

Educational Barriers. Those who were most successful had the highest levels of education and skill. Those with a high school diploma fared better than those with a GED, and clients with a technical or two-year degree were the most successful in sustaining employment (10 percent vs. 4 percent). Conversely, a two-year follow-up study by MDRC found that 20 percent of the NEWWS program group members had not worked during the follow-up period (Martinson, 2000). Those who never worked during the follow-up period had relatively low levels of education. Only one half had a high school diploma or GED certificate, compared with almost three-quarters of those who worked more than 75 percent of the follow-up period. Those who never worked were also very likely to have low basic skills. Over 56 percent scored low on a basic test of literacy and math skills (compared to 38 percent of the most successful groups).

Personal Barriers. Finally, those who were most successful in sustaining employment had fewer personal barriers to employment compared to those who were least successful. There were significant differences between the two groups in the proportion who reported family or personal problems, family attachment (the preference to stay home with children rather than returning to work), and locus of control (the degree to which a person feels in control of her life) as measured in the Private Opinion Survey (Martinson, 2000).

Facilitators to Obtaining and Sustaining Employment

Not only were there barriers to employment, the same studies also documented the existence of a variety of conditions that facilitated job placement and retention.

Recent Work History. Compared to the least successful group, those who were most successful in sustaining employment were more than twice as likely to have a recent work history. There could be several reasons for this association, ranging from individual attitudes to prior familiarity with the requirements of a work environment. The former could predispose an individual towards leaving or remaining in a position, while the latter could ease an individual's transition into a new job. Other underlying conditions might also account for the correlation between one's previous, present and future work history.

Relative Earnings and Working Conditions. When those who have been more successful in sustaining employment after leaving welfare are compared to those who have been less successful, research has determined that the more successful, even in their initial jobs, took jobs with better wages, benefits and hours than did the less successful (Martinson, 2000). For example, the NEWWS evaluation in Portland found that a large impact on earnings and employment could be produced in part by encouraging individuals to take "good" jobs from the beginning. Working full-time compared with part-time (20 hours or less) and higher initial wages were associated with more success in sustaining employment (Martinson, 2000).

Child Care. A mother's ability to find access to child care services has been found to be critical to job retention. In a study of the experiences of welfare recipients who find jobs, MDRC found that the group that was more successful in sustaining employment was more likely, when compared with less successful clients, to have used transitional child care payments made available by the state. At the same time, the more successful were also more likely to have paid out of pocket for child care (Martinson, 2000). Researchers argued that this could be because those who paid out of pocket worked and earned more than those not in regular employment or those who worked part-time, so the ability to find child care may be the result of an interaction effect with relative earnings and work conditions. There were no major differences across the groups in the extent to which they experienced child care problems that caused them to be absent or late for work.

Similarly, a review by MDRC of the Los Angeles Jobs-First GAIN Evaluation revealed that unreliable child care arrangements caused many members of the experimental group to miss or be late for work (Freedman, et al., 2000). This research suggested that welfare recipients with problems involving access to child care and/or transportation may benefit from access to post-employment services to increase job retention, and intensive case management services once they are employed. This type of social support also has a positive impact on parenting (Andresen and Telleen, 1992).

Health Insurance. In a study of the experiences of welfare recipients who found jobs, it was found that in the groups which were most successful in sustaining employment through the two-year follow-up after initial employment, twice as many had employer-provided medical insurance in their initial job compared to those who were least successful (44 percent vs. 17 percent). The group that was most successful was also over twice as likely to have other employer benefits such as paid sick time and vacation leave (Martinson, 2000).

The same study showed that those who were able to sustain employment were almost twice as likely to use transitional Medicaid at some point during the two-year follow-up period, when compared to women who were least successful in sustaining employment (47 percent vs. 26 percent). Transitional Medicaid was available to a client independent of her previous work experience or job skills. The researchers concluded that transitional Medicaid does appear to be an important factor in sustaining employment. Regardless of whether the health insurance was public or private, over 75 percent of the most successful group were covered by health insurance at the end of the two-year follow-up period compared to 30 percent for the least successful group.

AFTER TANF: THE ILLINOIS JOB ADVANTAGE PROGRAM

The Illinois Job Advantage Program ("Program") was a state-funded welfare-to-work program for public aid recipients designed to help the Illinois Department of Public Aid implement PRWORA and to assist the movement of welfare recipients into jobs. The State of Illinois elected to use an intensive case management approach for hard-to-place welfare clients during the first years of welfare reform in Illinois, and the Program was intended to provide this to their clients.

Social service agencies with a history of job training applied for state funds under the Program. The state then contracted with these agencies to provide case management, job training, job search, job placement and employment services. Social service agencies with Program funding received referrals from local offices of the Illinois Department of Public Aid (IDPA) to provide short-term job training, job search skills, job placement, and support services for welfare recipients. In this particular case management program, IDPA gave the agencies the hardest-to-place clients.

The Clients

The clients were primarily African-American women, 18-40 years old, with children. The majority had completed 8-9th grade and had a reading level of grade 7.1, were unmarried and lived in public housing near downtown Chicago or on the South Side or West Side. According to the reports of the case management agencies, 98 percent of the clients were females with children. Many of the women with children had three or more children. A small number had children who were involved in the state's foster care system and were in the process of regaining custody.

The Community-Based Agencies

At the beginning of the Program there were four agencies in one particular region of the city. Each of the agencies had a history in the community. The agencies serve some of the most distressed neighborhoods in the city (see Table 1).

One of the agencies was a small community-based agency where the executive director was a social worker. Consistent with a social work model, the staff were expected to assume multiple roles within the organization, and staff were expected to participate in weekly meetings to discuss each client's needs. A second agency was much larger and had a long history of helping the disabled. It incorporated the job placement program into its own department of adult rehabilitative services, which also provided mental health, substance abuse and domestic violence services. This agency made its job placement clients eligible for all other services within the organization. The third agency is a large, well-established community organization whose historical mission was to combine community development with economic empowerment. The organization originated in response to urban renewal programs that

TABLE 1. Illinois Job Advantage Community Areas Served

Community Area	1990 Population	% Having Female Heads	Median Household Income	% Unem- ployed	# Day Care Providers	Spaces
			Agency A			
Auburn Park/ Gresham	59,808	42	$27,547	16	17	1061
Woodlawn	27,473	57	$13,680	24	11	761
Bronzeville/ Douglas	30,652	66	$12,993	18	7	454
Englewood	48,434	59	$13,243	27	3	126
			Agency B			
Roseland	56,493	39	$28,601	18	14	N/A
Auburn Park	59,808	42	$27,547	16	17	N/A
Englewood	48,434	59	$13,243	27	3	126
			Agency C			
Grand Blvd	35,897	60	$7,146	34	17	1089
Kenwood	18,587	34	$22,808	6	5	290
Oakland	8,197	77	$5,909	45	8	361
Englewood	48,434	5959	$13,243	27	3	126
			Agency D			
Woodlawn	27,473	57	$13,680	24	11	761
Oakland	8,197	77	$5,909	45	8	361

threatened to displace community residents. The fourth agency specialized in job training and drug rehabilitation.

Agency Staff

Staff interviewed at the community-based agencies had a bachelors, masters, or equivalent college degree. The staff had experience in social work, career services, job placement and teaching within the community college system, the Illinois Department of Children and Family Services and rehabilitative services.

Staffing models varied at each agency. At one agency each staff member had familiarity with multiple roles within the agency so the agency could continue to function if other staff members were absent or they had to assume other responsibilities. At another agency different individuals served as job trainers in the job training component, job counselors for the clients' job search activities, and, after job placement, as job coaches and mentors.

Implementation

Each of the agencies had the following components in their case management programs.

Intake and Assessment of Clients. States were required by federal law to make an initial assessment of recipients' skills. Therefore each agency administered tests of their clients' reading and math skills at the time of enrollment. The results were used to develop a job training and job search plan for each client.

Some client characteristics made the transition from welfare to work particularly challenging. A great number of Program clients sent to the agencies from IDPA offices had no high school diploma or GED. Of those, a number were functionally illiterate, not being able to read or write well. Though the majority had completed 8th or 9th grade, some dropped out of school as early as the 6th grade. After case managers tested the reading and writing skills of the clients they made referrals for clients that let them be placed in jobs according to their reading ability.

Client Education and Skills Training. The Program provided up to six weeks of job skills training related to employment. Within the four agencies most job skills training was provided in the areas of hospitality (hotel and restaurant), security, computers and home health aide. The computer classes were offered daily for six weeks and were always filled.

Job Search Support. Federal law allows up to six weeks of job search activities (no more than four consecutive weeks) to count as work activities. In the Program many clients participated in a structured, directed job search. Some employers came on site to interview clients. Prior to on-site interviews with employers the agencies helped clients complete job applications resumes.

Staff found it absolutely necessary to teach hard-to-place clients effective job search behaviors. The staff took clients to job fairs, helped them fill out applications and stayed with them throughout the event. While at a job fair agency staff would walk clients through the job search process and talk with clients as they were doing it. If an interview resulted staff members took their clients to the job interview.

In order to create a supportive environment for the job search, the agencies offered job clubs. One of the agencies had a job club which met twice a week from 10:00 a.m. to 1:00 p.m.; clients were expected to stay with the job club until they were employed. Since clients had to be actively engaged in searching for work in order to receive welfare benefits, the agency felt that, in addition to meeting with a job counselor and searching want ads in the agency's office, it was important to meet as a women's support group to share strategies and gather information.

Prior to job interviews staff at the agencies coached clients on how to approach a job interview. This included role playing and videotaping. In addition, there was a video covering topics such as how and when to sit down at an interview, how to dress for an interview and other ways to make an interview more effective. To give just one example, the videos emphasized the importance of looking directly at a hiring manager, rather than looking down or looking away.

Appropriate dress for a job interview was discussed. Some agencies went further and gave their clients a complete interview outfit compiled by one of the cooperating social service agencies. An interview outfit included a dress, shoes, a purse, hose and a coat.

Support Services: Child Care. Because access to child care has been shown to be an important facilitator to sustained employment, PRWORA included funding for child care. In the Illinois Job Advantage program child care was an important consideration during the mother's job search. One of the agencies provided supervised child care on the premises, which meant that mothers could bring their children to the case management agency during their training and job search. In other instances the agency paid for child care while the mothers conducted their job search. Once a mother obtained a job IDPA would subsidize her child care. The mother paid a small monthly fee to the child care agency and IDPA paid the rest. As one agency staff member said, "We refer them to Cook County Child Care resource referrals. We help them complete the referral forms. We provide them 30 days of child care payment before the Illinois Department of Human Services starts the subsidized child care."

Support Services: Substance Abuse. PRWORA contained provisions tailored to meet the needs of specific special populations, including substance abusers. Substance abusers convicted of drug-related felonies do not qualify for cash assistance. Nothing in federal law prohibits states from performing drug tests on recipients, or sanctioning recipients who test positive for use of controlled substances. In the Program, for clients who were homeless, or those with drug or alcohol abuse problems but who had no drug-related felonies, referral systems were put in place before they began their job search activities. Clients with substance abuse problems were referred to a treatment program by the agency, and agency staff continued follow-up with the substance abuse treatment program personnel to see if clients were continuing treatment. After the client had undergone treatment and was drug-free, then the client returned to the agency to begin a job search.

Agency and Client Cooperation. It was understood that not all clients would, in their initial effort at completing the program and finding paid employment through the Program, remain in full compliance with the requirements of the Program. For this reason a step-wise process of notification, sanction and "reconciliation" was set in place.

Program Outcomes

The study obtained data from the agencies for a nine-month period in the first year of the program, April through December, 1998. The agencies supplied the number of clients enrolled in the intensive case management upon referral from Public Aid Office, the number of clients who completed the orientation and job search, and those who were placed in jobs.

Program Completion and Job Placement. Agency A received over 1000 referrals from IDPA, of whom 730 enrolled. At one point over 200 referrals arrived in two weeks. This was far too many new clients to process in such a short time. After the first surge of new clients changes were made to the Program so local public aid offices would refer a more steady stream of clients to the agencies each month. By December, 1998, 204 clients of Agency A had completed the orientation, six weeks of job training and job search. During the same monitoring period Agency B staff received 336 new clients as part of the Program. Of these, 256 clients completed the orientation, six weeks of job training, and job search. The agency placed 59 welfare clients in jobs between September and December, 1998. At Agency C, 256 clients were enrolled on the basis of Program referrals, with 96 clients completing six weeks of job training and job placement and nine clients placed in jobs by December. At Agency D, 174 clients were enrolled between April and August. By December, 179 clients, enrolling at varying times, had completed the six weeks of job training and job search activities, and 63 clients had been placed in jobs. A full evaluation of job placement under this program is being conducted by the Illinois Department of Public Aid.

It is tempting to try to determine the effectiveness of the program by simply adding up these figures. This is not appropriate, because the numbers do not represent a true cohort. The figures are only tracking numbers for the first nine months, not final figures on completion and placement. Some clients who enrolled in the Program prior to April, 1998 may be included in the figures for completions and placements. Similarly, some clients who enrolled in the spring of 1998 only completed their participation in job placement activities and found work after December, 1998. For instance, Agency A, still trying to process the many hundreds who had suddenly descended on it, was only in the middle of training when the nine months came to an end and did not report placements at all. Nevertheless, there is a discernable "bulge in the snake," a quasi-cohort with most enrollments in the spring, most program completions in the summer, and most placements in the fall. In this light, it should be noted that, even within this small window, the three agencies that reported placements were able to place 25 percent of those who completed the program. This is one quarter of those women who were considered the most difficult to place among the public aid caseload.

Job Retention and Sustained Employment. In addition to placing clients in jobs, job retention was a very important issue in the Program and it was in an agency's best interests to follow up once a client was employed. The stated goal of the Illinois Job Advantage Program was for each client to remain on the job for at least 90 days. Although agencies were reimbursed for clients who enrolled and participated in the Program, the state did not make full and final payment for an agency's job retention and other case management activities until a client had been working at the same job for 90 days. If the client left the job on day 89 the agency was not paid for the 89 days of job retention supervision that the agency provided. The client then returned to the agency (or was sanctioned) and began the process of job search and job interviews all over again.

A job coach was necessary to help the client navigate the workplace. Case managers across all agencies reported that job retention was their biggest challenge. It was the case managers' perception that three consecutive months on the job was a challenge for a number of women. Among the factors cited was the perception of the workplace, the perception of workplace authority, and illnesses on the part of the client or members of the client's family. As case managers reported in one agency: "Now we focus more on retention. We introduced incentives, such as graduation ceremonies attended by family and friends to motivate and encourage clients. Graduation occurs after completing the job skills training, and again after job retention for 90 days." At another agency staffers stated that they developed a retention class to give encouragement. "The class lasts 3-4 hours. It covers job issues brought by clients. Some of the working clients are asked to talk with those who are not working yet."

UNDERSTANDING THE PROCESS
OF PROGRAM IMPLEMENTATION IN ILLINOIS

Four community-based social service agencies active in this part of Chicago formed a partnership in order to apply for a grant under the Program. The executive committee for the partnership then asked faculty at the University of Illinois at Chicago to conduct interviews that would elicit perceptions of the Program from members of the staff of each agency. This included descriptions of the program each agency had developed, how the program model had evolved and the program's implementation at each agency. It also included the frustrations the agencies' staff had experienced in implementing the program and how case managers had addressed the client needs that they saw. The agencies also asked the evaluators to identify each program's strengths and opportunities for improvement, and how each agency's program might learn from the others. The program directors and case managers then planned to incorporate findings into the program implementation in subsequent months.

METHOD

This project used a participatory action research model in which the community organizations worked with the researchers to identify the types of questions which needed to be addressed (Reason, 1988; Kelly, 1986; Trickett, 1984). The academic researchers gave feedback to the case managers on themes that emerged from transcripts and notes and had the participants review the themes with the intention of incorporating them into their work with clients.

Focus Groups

After the first year of the Program four focus groups were conducted with case managers during March and April, 1999. The focus groups were conducted at the site of the case management agency, one focus group at each site. Across the four agencies, 20 case managers participated (ranging from four to seven case managers at each site). The case managers were African-Americans who had been serving African-American clients.

The focus groups were conducted by the authors of this paper at the request of the agency directors. The focus group interviews asked agency staff to describe the implementation of the program at their site. An interview guide was prepared for each focus group. The interview guide consisted of open-ended questions highlighting the following: (1) process evaluation; (2) current issues facing implementation of the case management program; (3) current issues facing the clients in job search and employment retention; (4) the structure of the program at their site. The focus group sessions were transcribed and coded for themes. In this way researchers were able to identify commonalties across sites as well as unique differences in implementation between sites.

In addition to the focus groups with case managers, the authors conducted interviews with each agency's program director. The authors also attended a day-long retreat conducted for program directors and staff from all four agencies.

Finally, individual interviews and focus groups were complemented with two sources of statistical information: (1) neighborhood demographic data and (2) site enrollment and job placement data.

An Ecological Model

This study used an ecological model to define the themes that emerged from focus group participants. The social ecological model uses multiple levels of social context to describe the influences on an individual's behavior. These levels include family, friends, neighbors, the neighborhood institutions such as schools and churches, the workplace environment, the governmental institutions at all levels–state and federal. When we try to address the transition from welfare to work on the part of mothers with children, the themes which resulted from the focus groups are best explained by the ecology of this transition, which gives the themes a meaningful relation to each other.

FINDINGS

A number of themes about client transitions to work emerged from the case manager focus groups. The problem was not a lack of jobs or willing employers. Other significant barriers emerged instead. In what follows, direct quotes from interviews, focus groups, and the retreat are noted as such, while extracts from our field materials are simply placed in block format.

Major Life Transitions and Case Management

The case managers reported that intensive case management was appropriate because their clients were experiencing changes so enormous that individualized programs for action helped them better adapt to the new world in which they found themselves. Across participating agencies, staff report that the transition from welfare to work was in and of itself a major life transition. More than that, this major life transition affected, and was in turn affected by, every level of a client's social ecology. In the judgement of agency staff this made wrap-around case management the most appropriate approach, because it emphasizes individualized job preparation and includes a comprehensive system of referrals to support her transition to work.

When trying to understand the issues at play in the lives of their clients, six levels emerged as those that most affected, and were affected by, the transition from welfare to work.

Awareness of Changes

Staff across all agencies felt it would be helpful to clients to understand the original intent of public aid so clients could understand that they were not being "pushed off" or discriminated against. Staff shared the fact that public assistance was developed 60 years ago to help families through a short term of unemployment while searching for another job, and that citizens do not have an inalienable right to public aid. Nevertheless, many clients did not understand the context for the previous law or the consequences of changes in the law: "Some clients are in denial about the change in the welfare program and refuse to believe that aid is time limited." As a result, case managers sought to inform clients how their present circumstances fit into the history of public aid and introduce public aid recipients to the significance of the recent changes in the law: "In our program clients learn how they fit into the larger world and the big picture issues of welfare reform."

Work Environment

Case managers found a welfare recipient's view of the work environment to be an important factor in the client's motivation and ultimate success, particularly the client's previous experiences with employers, view of authority, skill in working with coworkers, and financial planning for how to handle the wages received.

View of the Workplace. Many staff found that among their clients the most educated and most experienced persons were often the most difficult to place. Previous negative experiences on the job, or difficulty with authority, could hinder client performance once they obtained a job.

> The person with previous bad experiences in a job can appear to know it all and based on their previous experience have a higher status. . . . Clients with low skills can be influenced negatively by those with more work experience and can easily assimilate the anger of those who have had unpleasant experiences in the work force. Therefore, a support group for people just entering the work force for the first time has to be conducted as a group separate from those who have had previous negative experiences.

On the other hand, staff found that clients with low skills could at times be an "open book." Clients just entering the job market were more open to ideas from job developers and case managers. They were often eager to learn and appreciated the help provided to them in finding a job.

Response to Authority. The client's view of authority in the workplace was seen as critical to success on the job. One agency hired peer coaches who could meet the client at the job site or after work. The job coaches had to be prepared to teach the client how to handle work relationships. They also found that they had to teach the client how to respond to hostility on the job and how to de-escalate a tense workplace situation.

> We point out that even after you are hired, your immediate boss might not like you. . . . The case manager needs to be accessible when the client is first employed. We can assist you to try to resolve the problem; we emphasize that we are there to support you after you are hired. Clients ask, "How do I deal with a demanding employer?" or "How do I manage my work time?" When the client reaches the point of frustration, the staff have to be there or the client will walk off the job.

Anticipation of Racism. Concerns about racism were another barrier which clients expressed to their case managers. Case managers stated that even though racism still exists, they did not want client perceptions of racism to be used as an excuse not to enter the job market. In the focus groups the case managers discussed the strategies they provided clients in order for them to deal with racism. They taught clients how to deal with situations where they have had disrespect directed toward them.

Expectations for Conduct at Work and How to Interpret the Conduct of Others. The agency case managers talked with clients about jobs and what it means to hold a job. "We discuss what to expect on the job and what employers will expect of them. We discuss that when on a job you have to follow some rules and regulations." Case managers felt that clients needed to gain an understanding of the work world. They reported working with clients so they could present themselves to others in the work setting in an appropriate and confident manner.

> For example, clients were taught that it was to be expected that an employer would ask, "Where do you want to be in five years?" The question was not to be interpreted as "getting in your business." Further, when you introduce yourself to an employer, it is expected that you give both first and last name, not just first name.
> Staff at another agency report discussing the importance of not responding with insubordination, absenteeism, or tardiness and discussed ways to handle multiple task assignments.

In a similar vein, clients needed to learn how to inform employers when they have a family emergency or illness.

> One client had been a consistent worker, punctual and on the job everyday. Then, her son got shot in the head and was hospitalized. The mother went to visit the son every day in the hospital instead of going to work. When the employer called the case management agency and inquired about the absenteeism of the employee, the case manager found that the mother had been afraid to tell the agency. So, the case manager indicated to the client that she needed to be forthright and inform the employer about the family tragedy and work through it with the employer rather than ignore it.

Clients needed information about their employer's intent, especially that the actions of employers are not necessarily meant to be abandonment or disrespect.

One woman who was employed as a security guard was believed to be promising and was transferred to another location where she could get a promotion. As she was waiting an hour for her interview, she interpreted it as abandonment and left the premises and quit the job in disappointment and frustration.

Instruction in the Rewards of Work. Finally, in addition to providing help in the specific problem areas that could provide barriers to employment, agency staff believed that it was important to give people a vision to take home with them. They felt it was important to give clients realistic themes of success.

> For example, staff try to help clients understand that once they get a job, then they can continue to another job they want, be able to dress the way they want, and even own a house. Staff shared anecdotes of success illustrating what other clients have achieved once they became employed.

How to plan for the client's financial future was discussed in realistic terms, including how to obtain a more secure financial status.

> Staff also provide workshops in which they present financial information on topics such as the earned income tax credit. . . . Staff provide information on home ownership and how to develop a workable plan so that one day they can own their own home. Staff give help with housing. "We give home ownership information and neighborhood housing."

Socialization to the work environment appeared to be critical to the success of clients. A positive attitude toward one's coworkers and boss, a protocol for handling negative events, and tactics for responding to their own family needs are among the factors which needed to be imparted in this welfare-to-work program.

Neighborhood Environment: Neighborhood Resources and Social Norms

As was seen in Table 1, the agencies were located in some of the most impoverished neighborhoods in Chicago. Many clients were not embedded in neighborhood networks where they could discuss work issues or receive support for their efforts. These neighborhoods had the fewest jobs among the neighborhoods of the city, the greatest number of unemployed individuals and the greatest number receiving welfare. These were also the neighborhoods with the highest density of public housing projects. Neighborhoods with high unemployment, in which many of one's neighbors do not leave for work everyday, will exercise a different influence than those where work is the norm. A majority of the clients lived in these housing projects.

Family Environment

Clients often had to deal with the reactions of their social networks, particularly their families, to their search for a job. For example, one staff member told the story of a client whose family members–including a mother or sister–discouraged her from obtaining a job.

> The people close to you don't mean you harm when they discourage you from obtaining a job. They just can't see you hurt. Why should you try this job search again when it causes you so much pain. However, with that attitude, they help you not help yourself. Because the job search and job loss have caused you pain in the past, your close friend or family member will worry about you and will discourage you from attempting something which causes you pain.

Clients often needed to renegotiate their family and work roles. For instance, clients were required to deal with the effect of work on their role as a parent.

> Work will change their lives at home. The mother has to get everyone in the household involved in the process of "me" working. Mothers have to reorganize time and tasks. Even the act of preparing a dinner is different when you are working. For example, the children all have to be involved in the steps necessary to produce the dinner. The children need to help with the laundry, sort clothes and then the mother can go to the park with the children or rent a video which they can watch together after all the chores have been completed. Parenting practices and parenting roles have to be renegotiated. The agency can refer mothers to support programs or discussion programs on parenting which are locally available.

Case managers also reported that they had to deal with domestic violence in order to help a woman get a job and stay on the job. As one of the life skills seminars offered during the job search process, one agency addressed responses to domestic violence.

Agency staffers responded to the clear effect family networks had on the transition from welfare to work by addressing the issue explicitly, by teaching clients how to respond to the concerns of family members and renegotiate their roles as necessary, and by offering clients sources of social reinforcement that were separate from and an alternative to social reinforcement from relatives who may have been barriers to a transition to work.

> Case managers report that the client needs to deal with her social support network. Case managers asked clients, "What does your family say about this?" Her network needs to be supportive of her job search and working. The agency attempts to encourage support for the client by recognizing her efforts at social gatherings and recognition ceremonies such as graduation (speeches, plaques, certificates).

The support provided by a family network is important to obtaining and retaining a job. Case managers found that support from a spouse was extremely important. Recognizing this fact, the intent of the new welfare law was to strengthen the father's role and provide support for fathers as well as mothers in obtaining work, and to enforce child support payments should the father leave.

Literacy and Education

Though literacy and education are important in keeping and retaining a job, the case managers did not have the resources to help their clients. One agency in particular reported that the majority of clients who came to their agency had no high school diploma or GED; a significant number were functionally illiterate, not being able to read or write well. Some dropped out of school as early as the 6th grade. This limited the number, quality and type of jobs available for that client. The issue of computer literacy was the focus of the job skill training at one of the agencies.

Participants in the focus groups suggested that, in actuality, the welfare clients referred to them as "Job Ready," as assessed by education and previous work experience, were often among the most difficult to place.

For example, the high school graduate who has had 3-4 previous jobs and has language skills and presents herself well, may be angry and have other emotional problems and may not want to work. This type of client requires a different approach than those who are eager to join the work force and haven't worked in the past. The educated client with emotional problems can be condescending in a group and present their anger and cynicism about the workplace to others.

In a seeming paradox, then, education could interact with other aspects of the client's social environment to produce barriers to employment that were even stronger than either would have been otherwise.

Emotional Environment

The interaction found between education and mental health was not at all unusual in this study. Staff found in general that the emotions held by their clients had a profound effect on the course of their clients through the programs offered by the agencies. Indeed, mental health problems were among the biggest barriers to job placement and retention.

Anger and Suspicion. Many came to the case management agencies angry and suspicious of the agency: "They come angry at the referral from public aid to our agency. When clients come they will often say, 'I don't know why I'm here.' It is necessary to challenge this. It is necessary to defuse the anger while also allowing clients a chance to vent."

Some staff reported that there were some clients who viewed the helpfulness of the agency as a weakness which was to be taken advantage of . . .

Clients would manipulate "the system" in place at the agency by selling the transportation bus tokens which they were given for job interviews and by skipping from program to program within the agency and from training program to training program to extend the time without a job.

Sometimes anger and suspicion would lead a client to sabotage a job interview.

For those clients who are told, "You can't go to an interview in jeans or take your kids with you," and then they do it and don't get the job. In those cases, we give them another chance. But if they break the next interview appointment or don't follow the interviewing rules, then we send them a reconciliation letter. Twenty-five percent of our cases end in reconciliation. If they don't respond to our letters and calls, we report the non-compliance to public aid and public aid stops their checks. When public aid stops the checks they come back to us and begin the job search cycle all over again.

Fortunately, often it was possible to gradually overcome negative emotions directed toward agency staff as progress was made each day in finding a job and the client began feeling more comfortable with this life transition. The thing that proved to help the most was implementing a plan and making progress toward finding a job.

Personal Sense of Control. In a study of welfare recipients who found jobs and were successful in sustaining employment for two years after initial job placement, Martinson (2000) found that 30 percent of those who never worked had a personal or family barrier and only 10 percent had a sense of personal control over one's life, compared with 17 percent of the more successful group.

This study also found that case managers at the agencies believed that a personal sense of control was important to address and develop in clients. Several staffers reported having to deal with excuses clients gave for not being able to find and keep a job. For example, in one agency, staff reported that they brought client excuses out into the open, confronting them, and then talking about the real issues that led to their child care or transportation problems. "The goal is to help empower the woman to manage the issues behind the excuses." One staff member described a continuum of moving through the job program that gives clients a gradually increasing sense of control. Staff also worked with clients to develop self-confidence, to fight the fear and take a risk. "This builds client self-esteem and empowers the client to achieve a sense of personal control over her situation."

Depression. In a study of 20 welfare-to-work programs conducted by MDRC the women who showed signs of depression at the start of the program were less able to capitalize on work to increase earnings. The researchers suggested that welfare administrators might need to implement different or more intensive treatments for depressed clients (Michalopoulos, Schwartz, & Adams-Ciardullo, 2000).

Staff also commented that they needed to work with the mothers' own feelings of depression and being overwhelmed because the mothers' depressed feelings will affect her child and the child's functioning.

The concerns expressed by staff are quite real. Research has found that maternal depression has strong effects on the behavioral and cognitive developmental outcomes of their children. Depressed mothers are more likely to exhibit less responsive or hostile, harsh parenting (McGroder, 2000). Whether the effect of depression on maternal employment is quite as strong remains an open question (see Hair, this volume, and cf. Martinson, 2000).

Resiliency: Ability to Respond to Setbacks. The client's belief in her ability to bounce back from setbacks during this major life change is critical. One case management agency found they had to view job search and job placement in the welfare-to-work context as not just looking for a job, but as a major life change that affected all aspects of the client's life. For this reason clients making the change from welfare to work often cycle in and out of jobs, and for a period may move from one job to another. This made learning how to bounce back from setbacks an important aspect of the welfare-to-work transition.

> For example, at one agency there was a 32-year-old client with five children who had never had a job. She went through the orientation and job search phase. She got a job and was so surprised. She felt extremely pleased. However, when she lost the job through cutbacks, she felt humiliated and embarrassed. She didn't want to come back to the agency, which is the normal course, and go through the job search again. When the employer informed the agency that she had been terminated, one of the agency staff wrote her a letter and expressed how difficult it was to lose a job and invited her to come back and start the process again. She didn't respond. As a result of not responding and going back on welfare, she was using up her time-limited welfare payments. The staff tracked down a family member from her contact sheet and that family member talked with her. It turns out that the client was devastated by the loss of the job and couldn't face anyone, let alone the agency which had helped her. Three weeks later the case management agency hired her to work as a mentor to TANF recipients to encourage and engage them in the job search process. Their former client is flourishing as their employee.

Further research is needed to understand the full impact of mental health problems in limiting the effectiveness of welfare-to-work programs. It is clear, though, that additional efforts need to be made to provide increased availability and accessibility to mental health services for low-income persons.

Summary

Agency staff responsible for implementing the program felt that an intensive case management approach was appropriate in this context, both because the movement from welfare to work was a major life transition in its own right and because it interacted with other life transitions being faced by their clients. Success was facilitated by assistance on the part of those with knowledge about work and other resources that could be brought to bear on the process. In addition, agency staff found that a mother's transition was dependent upon support from at least six distinct levels: (1) her awareness of the requirements of the law; (2) the environmental context and social norms common in her neighborhood; (3) family support, family structure and family expectations; and individual factors such as: (4) emotional well-being; (5) literacy and education; and (6) appropriate expectations of the work environments.

DISCUSSION

Findings from this study demonstrate that the transition from welfare to work is a complex process, frought with many barriers along the way. The programs described in this study sought to create a capacity for an adaptive response to changed circumstances.

Further, as mothers with young children make this transition, these findings support the importance of intensive case management in assisting them to shape adaptive responses. Though funding from the State of Illinois for intensive case management in helping clients transition from welfare to work is no longer available, it remains the case that help with the transition to work is best done by agencies with sustained involvement and contact with their clients, such as preschools, Head Start centers, social service agencies, etc. A number of the strategies reported by case managers participating in these focus groups would be useful to other social service and educational programs that work with clients who are parents.

The major findings of this study can be applied to helping the client transition to work. The ecological framework is particularly useful in providing structure to the emotional support that must be given to women entering the work force. In particular, women needed information and guidance regarding the six dimensions of their social environment that emerged with such salience: (1) changes in the laws and regulations regarding public aid; (2) the work environment; (3) support from neighborhood resources; (4) family support; (5) personal literacy, job-specific skills and education; and (6) emotional barriers such as anger, depression, and a personal sense of control.

Further, it appears that as the welfare-to-work clients represented by this population are stabilized in the work force, they could also benefit from the intensive strategies found so effective in the JOBS program: information on budgeting and financial planning, including financial planning for housing, food and other daily life strategies. Training in the practical life skills necessary to make a go of it in the world of work should not be underestimated. It also helps for agencies to have experience in placing people who have learning disabilities and/or low functional literacy.

In addition to practical life skills, those agencies with greater success–more clients placed in jobs and more clients retained in jobs for at least three months–had access to comprehensive support services for clients, including mental health counseling, job skills training, and motivational and social skills training.

There may be a simple reason that greater success was associated with greater coordination and collaboration among community agencies serving low-income women transitioning from welfare to work, including mental health, substance abuse, domestic violence, and educational programs. These support services, far from being secondary, may have acted to increase employment. Efforts to cultivate the personal resilience of clients may be important for the long-term process of movement from welfare to work, as in so many other of life's challenges.

Previous research has found that the first job sets the client on a trajectory that will continue for years to come. Those previous welfare clients who are most likely to sustain employment and increase earnings are those whose first job had a livable wage and provided benefits. The intensive case management approach as reported in these focus groups is the type of job search and job placement program that is most likely to prepare a client for better jobs when she leaves welfare and therefore sustain employment.

NOTE

1. See http://www.access.gpo.gov/congress/wm015.txt

REFERENCES

Andresen, P. & Telleen, S. (1992). The relationship between social support and maternal behaviors and attitudes: A meta-analytic review. *American Journal of Community Psychology, 20*, 753-774.

Danziger, S., Corcoran, M., Danziger, S., Heflin, C., Kalil, A., Levine, J., Rosen, D., Seefeldt, K., Siefert, K., & Tolman, R. (2002). *Barriers to the employment of welfare recipients*. Michigan: University of Michigan, Poverty Research & Training Center.

Freedman, S., Friedlander, D., Hamilton, G., Rock, J., Mitchell, M., Nudelman, J., Schweder, A., & Storto, L. (2000). *National evaluation of welfare-to-work strategies. Evaluating alternative welfare-to-work approaches: Two-year impacts for eleven programs*. Washington, DC: U.S. Department of Health and Human Services, Administration for Children and Families, Office of the Assistant Secretary for Planning and Evaluation; and U.S. Department of Education, Office of the Under Secretary and Office of Vocational and Adult Education.

Illinois Department of Public Aid (1997). *State of Illinois: Plan for temporary assistance for needy families*. Springfield, IL: Illinois Department of Public Aid.

Kelly, J. (1986). Context and process: An ecological view of the interdependence of practice and research. *American Journal of Community Psychology 14*, 581-599.

Kelly, J. G., Ryan, A. M., Altman, B. E., & Stelzner, S. P. (2000). Understanding and changing social systems: An ecological view. In J. Rapaport & E. Seidman (Eds.), *Handbook of community psychology* (pp. 133-159). New York: Kluwer Academic/Plenum Publishers.

Lennon, M. C., Blome, J., & English, I. (2001). *Depression and low-income women: Challenges for TANF and welfare-to-work policies and programs*. Research Forum on Children, Families and the New Federalism. New York: National Center for Children in Poverty, Columbia University.

Martinson, K. (2000). *The national evaluation of welfare-to-work strategies: The experience of welfare recipients who find jobs*. Washington, DC: U.S. Department of Health and Human Services, Administration for Children and Families, Office of the Assistant Secretary for Planning and Evaluation; and U.S. Department of Education, Office of the Under Secretary and Office of Vocational and Adult Education.

Michalopoulos, C., & Schwartz, D. (2000). *What works best for whom: Impacts of 20 welfare-to-work programs by subgroup: The national evaluation of welfare-to-work strategies*. New York, NY: Manpower Demonstration Research Corporation.

Reason, P. (Ed.). (1988). *Human inquiry in action: Developments in new paradigm research*. London: Sage Publications.

Telleen, S. (1990). Parental beliefs and help-seeking in mothers' use of a community-based family support program. *Journal of Community Psychology, 18*, 264-276.

Trickett, E. J. (1984). Toward a distinctive community psychology: An ecological metaphor for the conduct of community research and the nature of training. *American Journal of Community Psychology 12*, 261-280.

Welfare, Work and Well-Being Among Inner-City Mothers

Kathleen S. Crittenden
Seijeoung Kim
Kaoru Watanabe
Kathleen F. Norr

The University of Illinois at Chicago

SUMMARY. Family life cycle influences maternal labor force participation and well-being. We model the employment status and well-being of minority, low-income women, recruited during late pregnancy, when their children are 12, 24 and 36 months old. Non-time-varying predictors include mother's ethnicity, age, parity, education, recent household employment experience, birth cohort and initial welfare participation. Time and later fertility are nested within individuals. Welfare participation declined from 80% to 46% by 36 months; employment increased from 12% to 44%, and full-time employment from 6% to 29%. Likelihood of work-

Address correspondence to: Kathleen S. Crittenden, Department of Sociology, M/C 312, University of Illinois at Chicago, 1007 W. Harrison Street, Chicago, IL 60607.

This research was funded by the Agency for Health Care and Policy Research (Grant HS 07624), the National Institute of Nursing Research (Grant NR 04316), and the University of Illinois at Chicago (Great Cities Institute, Campus Research Board, Center for Research on Women and Gender, and Dean's Fund of the College of Nursing). The REACH/Futures intervention was funded by the American Academy of Pediatrics, the Division of Maternal and Child Health of the Department of Health and Human Services, the University of Illinois Hospital, and the Irving Harris Foundation.

[Haworth co-indexing entry note]: "Welfare, Work and Well-Being Among Inner-City Mothers." Crittenden, Kathleen S. et al. Co-published simultaneously in *Journal of Prevention & Intervention in the Community* (The Haworth Press, Inc.) Vol. 23, No. 1/2, 2002, pp. 41- 64; and: *The Transition from Welfare to Work: Processes, Challenges, and Outcomes* (ed: Sharon Telleen, and Judith V. Sayad) The Haworth Press, Inc., 2002, pp. 41- 64. Single or multiple copies of this article are available for a fee from The Haworth Document Delivery Service [1-800-HAWORTH, 9:00 a.m. - 5:00 p.m. (EST). E-mail address: getinfo@haworthpressinc.com].

41

ing was enhanced by high school education and household work experience, but hindered by repeat pregnancy. Among women initially on welfare, working increased over time; among non-welfare recipients, African Americans were more likely to work. When causally prior predictors were controlled, working full-time decreased difficult life circumstances but employment did not affect depression. Evaluations of welfare policy should consider life-cycle events, focusing on small increments of time around the birth of a child. *[Article copies available for a fee from The Haworth Document Delivery Service: 1-800-HAWORTH. E-mail address: <getinfo@haworthpressinc.com> Website: <http://www. HaworthPress.com> © 2002 by The Haworth Press, Inc. All rights reserved.]*

KEYWORDS. Low-income women, life cycle, employment, well-being

INTRODUCTION

Poverty has been an intractable problem in the United States, especially for minority mothers and their children. In the 1980s and 1990s about 20% of all children were poor, almost half of these extremely poor (Annie E. Casey Foundation, 1999), but poverty rates remain higher for minorities and for households headed by women (U. S. Census, 1990). Over 40% of African American and Hispanic children under age six live in poverty (45% and 42%, respectively). Over half of all persons in African American and Hispanic female-headed families (53% and 61%, respectively) are poor. The Aid to Families of Dependent Children (AFDC) rolls increased after 1962 and jumped by 29% between 1989 and 1993, peaking at over 13.6 million in 1993 (Joseph, 1999). With the cost of entitlements soaring and public support declining, welfare policy has, since 1988, focused on moving AFDC recipients from welfare to self-sufficiency through work.

Most families on welfare have children of preschool age (Burtless, 1997; Henle & Ali, 1996). Little is known, though, about the activities of poor mothers as they negotiate the changing responsibilities of caring for and financially supporting their families as their children progress from infancy through the formative early years. Does taking welfare during times of maximal family responsibilities inhibit poor mothers' likelihood of working in the long term? Will working improve their life circumstances?

The research reported here is based on data from a panel of 435 minority, low-income women in inner-city Chicago, recruited during late pregnancy in 1993-1996 and followed until their babies reached the age of three. The panel was ongoing in 1996 when the Personal Responsibility and Work Opportunity Reconciliation Act (PRWORA), intended to "end welfare as we know it," was signed into law by then-President Clinton. These mothers, some on welfare, some working, but all poor, would be among those most affected by welfare reform. We realized that the information already being collected from them offered a valuable window through which to observe prospectively the strategies that families in poverty use to balance family and economic responsibilities during a dynamic period both in the family cycle and in the welfare policy environment.

The research has three objectives: (1) to describe patterns of welfare participation, work and fertility among these mothers from pregnancy through their babies' first three years; (2) to explain their work participation over this period on the basis of personal and household characteristics, initial welfare participation and subsequent fertility; and (3) to consider the impact of employment on their personal well-being.

BACKGROUND AND HYPOTHESES

Factors that Influence Employment

According to the human capital perspective (Becker, 1993; Bourdieu, 1986; Harris, 1993, 1996), a woman's likelihood of labor force participation is a function of factors that influence the costs and benefits of, and barriers to, working. These include human capital and other personal characteristics, events in the family/life cycle and factors in the external environment.

Women with greater investments in human capital, such as education, work experience and job skills, will be more successful in the labor market. Education is the most important form of human capital. In addition to providing the knowledge and skills required by a specific job or the economy, education is general and transferable, promoting an individual's ability to adjust to new tasks. Socialization through schooling also fosters personality traits that help the individual fit into different work settings. Finally, employers use education as evidence that an applicant possesses skills, trainability and desirable attitudes (Holzer, 1996). Work experience develops work skills and knowledge of workplace norms (Harris, 1993) and, to employers, signals commitment to the labor force (Holzer, 1996). Work experience on the part of other household members contributes capital resources as well.

Longitudinal surveys spanning several decades have established the influence of education and work experience on the success of low-income women in negotiating the welfare-to-work process, that is, in finding work, leaving welfare and/or remaining off welfare (Brooks & Buckner, 1996; Danziger et al., 2000; Ellwood, 1988; Harris, 1993, 1996; Illinois Department of Human Services [IDHS], 2000b; Kalil et al., 1998; Martinson, 2000). Conversely, low levels of education (less than a high school education) and work experience reduce both employment and earnings.

Investments in family may compete with investments in human capital. Early childbearing may interfere with one's investment in education, job training or work experience, while subsequent fertility and parenting responsibilities may further limit a woman's ability to work. Research has documented that pregnancy has strong short-term effects on women's participation in the work force. In a study that tracked employment in a national sample of U. S. women from one year before birth until two years following birth (Waite, Haggstrom & Kanouse, 1985), 70% of the women were employed 12 months before birth. Likelihood of being employed decreased markedly late in pregnancy, reaching a low point (20%) in the month of the birth. Employment rates rose after delivery, but not to the initial, pre-birth levels. Using similar methodology, Ortiz and Fennelly (1988) tracked employment trajectories around the time of a first birth, by ethnicity, for a national sample of women who had given birth before age 22. Although African American and Mexican American women had lower levels of working than white women, the three groups had similar trajectories around the time of birth.

Some researchers have reported lower employment levels associated with early childbearing (Brooks & Buckner, 1996; Danziger et al., 2000) and with having very young children. Additional children increase the need for a mother's financial contribution, but also the relative value of her productivity at home. Harris (1993, 1996) found that women with larger families are less likely to leave welfare through work and have more welfare recidivism. There is a wage-penalty of about 7% per child associated with motherhood, which reduces to about 4% when personal and job characteristics are controlled (Budig & England, 2001).

Since the mid-1980s the major debate in poverty policy has concerned whether receiving welfare perpetuates poverty by discouraging work (Harris, 1993). When earnings are balanced by equivalent cuts in welfare benefits (and often elimination of medical coverage), women have little incentive to seek work. Yet longitudinal studies have documented substantial work activity among welfare recipients over the past two decades (Brooks & Buckner, 1996; Harris, 1993; Spalter-Roth, Burr, Hartmann & Shaw, 1995). Throughout this period, a sizeable proportion of single mothers have combined welfare and work or cycled between them. One study (Pavetti, 1996) found that welfare recipients left jobs at higher rates than non-recipients with comparable education and family characteristics. No studies have examined the effect of welfare participation on working in the context of the parenting life cycle.

External factors that influence employment prospects include the economy and labor market conditions, welfare policy and such resources and barriers as the availability of child care and transportation. In general, a robust economy will facilitate the welfare-to-work process by enhancing both wages and the supply of jobs. By reducing demand-side constraints to employment, a strong economy increases the relative importance of supply-side constraints related to the woman's human capital investments.

What kinds of work do poor women do? Access to most entry-level jobs available to workers without a college degree requires credentials that many welfare recipients lack: a high school diploma, work experiences and references (Holzer, 1996). In addition, most of these jobs require occupants to perform on a daily basis one or more of the following tasks: reading and writing paragraphs, dealing with customers, doing arithmetic and using computers.

When welfare recipients take jobs they work in the service sector, in sales, in manufacturing and as laborers (Brooks & Buckner, 1996; Danziger et al., 2000; Harris, 1993; IDHS, 2000b), depending on the structure of the local economy. Within those sectors they work primarily in low wage jobs such as cashier or food service worker. Often the work is part time and/or intermittent. Research has shown consistently that the wages these women earn are insufficient to raise their families above poverty level (Brooks & Buckner, 1996; Danziger et al., 2000; Harris, 1993; Joseph, 1999). This has been true even for women participating in formal job-preparation programs (Freedman et al., 2000; IDHS, 2000b; Martinson, 2000).

The welfare policy context also influences the reward/cost tradeoffs between work and family responsibilities. In particular, a poor woman's likelihood of working is affected by the prevailing availability and level of welfare benefits in a particular setting, as well as the requirements or incentives for recipients to work. Without work requirements or incentives to work, a more generous welfare policy may be associated with lesser work force participation.

The effort to "reform" welfare as we had known it began with the Family Support Act of 1988, which established the Job Opportunities and Basic Skills Training (JOBS) program. To reduce welfare dependency JOBS emphasized education and training, job placement, child care and other supportive services.

Historically, Illinois welfare programs have nearly always included work and vocational training. Starting in 1993 the state participated in a welfare demonstration project, Work Pays, that incorporated several key JOBS provisions: work, education and training requirements, wage subsidies and time-limited assistance in which the "clock" stops during periods of employment (Lewis, George & Puntenney, 1999; U. S. Department of Health and Human Services [USDHHS], 1996). The program encouraged employment by allowing welfare recipients who worked to keep two out of three dollars they earned until they reached the poverty level (about three times the amount of the AFDC grant). In 1995, the state added a parental responsibility demonstration program that denied benefits for additional children (USDHHS, 1996). The AFDC caseload in Illinois peaked at 710,000 in 1994, then began to decline (Joseph, 1999). Under Work Pays, the proportion of AFDC recipients with earned income increased from 8% in 1993 to over 27% in 1997 (Lewis et al., 1999).

In 1997 PRWORA eliminated AFDC and the JOBS program, replacing them with Temporary Assistance for Needy Families (TANF). The legislation eliminated family assistance as an entitlement, mandating work requirements for recipients and lifetime limits for receipt of benefits. States were given considerable discretion in defining allowable work activities and other program details. By early 1997 AFDC caseloads across the nation had declined by 20% from their 1993 peak, and the decline was accelerated under TANF. The number of recipients declined by 37% from August 1996 to December 1998. However, most families who have left the welfare rolls remain below the poverty line, moving from welfare to the ranks of the working poor (Joseph, 1999).

Like Work Pays, the Illinois TANF plan has been designed to reward and reinforce work efforts on the part of recipients (Illinois Department of Public Aid [IDPA], 1997; IDHS, 2000b; Joseph, 1999; Lewis et al.,

1999). Non-pregnant women are considered "available to work." The state has continued the earnings disregard that reduces TANF grants by only $1 for each $3 earned. It has adopted a five-year lifetime limit for receipt of benefits, but unlike most states, Illinois does not apply the limit to recipients who work a minimum number of hours. The state policy provides for child care subsidies along with other supportive services for working recipients, and extends these and medical services to those transitioning off TANF. By 1998, one year after implementation of TANF, the TANF caseload in Illinois was down 42% from the 1994 peak, but this was still the third highest TANF caseload of any state (IDHS, 2000b; Joseph, 1999).

AFDC/TANF dollar grants in Illinois have become increasingly less generous over time, from 62% of the standard of need in 1982 to 38% in 1997, and they are low compared with most other midwestern states (Lewis et al., 1999). The obvious inadequacy of these grants to meet a family's needs, before and after implementation of TANF, and the absence of time limits for working recipients should make working relatively attractive to an Illinois welfare recipient. Theoretically a woman could increase her family income up to threefold by combining welfare with suitable work, to reach the poverty level. However, given her qualifications and the work available (even in a robust economy), she has little likelihood of escaping poverty through work.

Availability of affordable child care and transportation in the vicinity also affects a woman's employment prospects. Despite provisions for child care subsidies, child care was a major barrier to employment for mothers of young children in the pre-TANF period because of the shortage of licensed child care services in Illinois (Henle & Ali, 1996; IDPA, 1995). Few existing child care facilities were able to accommodate the odd-hour shifts typical of many entry-level jobs (Henle & Kinsella, 1996). Under TANF, the state has moved to open new child care facilities with more flexible hours in an attempt to meet the greatly expanded demand for services (IDHS, 2000a). However, in the early TANF period, access to child care has remained a significant barrier to employment for mothers of infants and toddlers in Illinois (IDHS, 2000a, 2000b) and other states (e.g., Danziger et al., 2000).

There often is a spatial mismatch between available jobs and available low-skill workers, and automobile ownership is low among low-income, inner-city families (Carlson & Theodore, 1997). As a result, transportation to work and to child care has been a consistent obstacle to maternal employment in Illinois throughout our study period (e.g., Henle & Kinsella, 1996).

Based on a human capital and family life event perspective and the literature we have reviewed, we expect that the labor force participation of inner-city mothers will, in the three years after giving birth, be affected in the following ways. The likelihood of employment should be enhanced by education and household work experience, but be lower for teen mothers, multiparous women and those on welfare around the time of birth. Employment rates should be higher for mothers whose babies were younger in 1997 when TANF was implemented. Finally, labor force participation should increase as the baby ages and decrease with subsequent pregnancies.

Work and Well-Being

For the mothers of young children, having a job involves balancing family and work roles. Playing multiple roles is a potential source of stress as well as a source of gratification and resource for coping with stress (Aneshensel, Frerichs & Clark, 1981; Thoits, 1991). To the extent that the different roles compete for a woman's time and resources and involve contradictory role expectations, they may detract from her psychological well-being. This possibility may be exacerbated for poor women. On the other hand, multiple roles can also be gratifying and enhance psychological health.

In a cross-sectional study based on a national sample of adult women in the U. S. in 1992, Cho (1999) found that, whether they resided with a male partner or not, mothers employed outside the home had lower levels of depressive symptoms than mothers who did not work. This result suggests that, for mothers in general, the psychological benefits associated with working may outweigh the costs. However, for mothers in poverty employment may offer fewer rewards–either financial or psychological–and result in more stress from role conflict than would be true for a broader cross-section of mothers.

Although the primary purpose of recent welfare reforms was to trim the AFDC/TANF rolls, the rationale offered for both the Family Support Act of 1988 and PRWORA emphasized the benefits to recipients: Work enhances psychological well-being as well as financial stability.

Given the financial incentives attached to work in Illinois welfare policy, we expect working to lessen a woman's difficult life circumstances. In addition, we tentatively propose that she should be less depressed during periods of employment.

METHOD

Participants

Data for this study are taken from a panel of women recruited to a randomized trial of a community-based parenting intervention program (Boyd, Norr & Nacion, 2001). A total of 617 women were recruited in late pregnancy from two prenatal clinics of the University of Illinois at Chicago Medical Center (UIMC) during the period from November 1993 to September 1996. The sample was designed to be approximately two-thirds African American and one-third Latina. All were low-income, inner city women who lived in community areas with high infant mortality served by UIMC. Recruitment criteria verified from the medical record included the following: eligible for Medicaid or state supplemental health insurance (income under 150% of poverty); address in designated community areas at the time of recruitment; medically low-risk; and experiencing a low risk pregnancy with no evidence of current drug use.

Our research followed the mother until her baby reached the age of three. In addition to the initial intake interview, this paper uses data from interviews conducted at 12, 24 and 36 months after the baby's birth. Retention was 82% over 12 months and 72% over 24 months. The analysis was limited to the 435 respondents self-identified as African American or Mexican American (discarding the small numbers of other Latinas and respondents who did not reside with their babies) who had been interviewed at intake, 12 months and 24 months. We attempted 36-month interviews only with the 377 women among this group whose babies were born after May 1994. An 82% response rate among these resulted in 310 36-month interviews.

Measures

Independent variables. Background characteristics were assessed in the intake interview (except as noted for initial welfare participation). These included ethnicity (African American vs. Mexican American); age (teen vs. 20+); parity (multiparous vs. primiparous); and education (at least high school or G.E.D. vs. less). We used three measures of household employment experience (each coded as yes/no): whether another household member had worked in the last 12 months; whether the respondent had worked in the last 12 months; and whether she had ever worked for six months.

Birth cohort reflected the baby's birth date, taken from birth records. Respondents in Cohort 1 had babies born between November 1993 and June 1995, so when TANF was implemented in Illinois in July 1997 their babies were already two or three years old. Cohort 2 had given birth July 1995 to August 1996; their babies were in their second year as TANF went into effect. Initial welfare participation was coded 1 (yes) if the respondent reported receiving AFDC at intake or within six months after giving birth, otherwise the response was coded as 0.

Group assignment in the randomized trial and two measures of household composition–co-residence with a mother (or mother figure) and co-residence with a male partner-were not related to any outcome in this paper, so we omitted these variables from all analyses.

Outcomes. Repeated measures of outcomes with respect to fertility, work, welfare and well-being were taken at intake and at 12, 24 and 36 months after the initial birth. A repeat pregnancy at any given wave was a current pregnancy or birth within the previous 12 months. Note that, given appropriate timing, the same pregnancy could to be recorded at two subsequent waves. We measured current employment two ways: first, whether the respondent worked at all and second, whether she worked full-time (each yes/no). For the 12-, 24- and 36-month waves, welfare participation reflected whether respondent reported current participation in AFDC/TANF at any given time.

We used two measures of well-being or lack thereof at each wave: difficult life circumstances and depression. The Difficult Life Circumstances Scale (DLC) (Barnard, 1989) is a count of 28 binary items reflecting chronic, current stressors that the respondent might be experiencing (e.g., lack of money for bills). The test-retest correlation between intake and 12 months was .50 for our respondents. Depression was measured with the Center for Epidemiological Studies Depression Scale (CES-D), a 20-item self-report scale assessing the frequency of depressive symptoms experienced in the previous week (range: 0-60) (Radloff, 1977; Weissman, Sholomskas, Pottenger, Prusoff & Locke, 1977). It has well-established concurrent and discriminant validity for community and patient populations and reliability as assessed by internal consistency (Boyd, Weissman, Thompson & Myers, 1982; Orme, Reis & Herz, 1986; Radloff & Locke, 1986; Santor, Zuroff, Ramsay, Cervantes & Palacios, 1995). Referral for professional evaluation is recommended for scores of 16 or higher (Myers & Weissman, 1980; Roberts & Vernon, 1983). The CES-D has been used successfully in studies of depression in new mothers (e.g., Leathers, Kelley & Richman, 1997; Logsdon, McBride & Birkimer, 1994). For our sample, Cronbach alpha reliability coefficients ranged from .85 to .87 within waves, and the test-retest correlation between intake and 12 months was .55.

ANALYSES AND RESULTS

Sample Characteristics

Two thirds (68.5%) of the study panel were African American and two thirds (66.0%) were in birth Cohort 1. At intake 39.1% were teens, 45.1% were multiparous, 52.4% lived with their mothers and 28.0% lived with male partners. About half (50.3%) had a high school degree or equivalent. Only one fourth (24.8%) had worked in the last 12 months, but over half (57.2%) had at least six months of work experience. Sixty-three percent lived in households in which another household member had worked in the last year.

Trends in Welfare, Work, Fertility and Well-Being

Our first research goal was to describe welfare, work and fertility over a three-year period for the sample. Table 1 summarizes these trajectories. Welfare participation, initially at 80%, declined as the babies grew older, dropping to 46% at 36 months. Over the three-year period the likelihood that someone in the household was working increased, from 60% to 76%. This trend was due to a 250% increase in employment activity on the part of the new mothers over time, from 12% at intake to 44% at 36 months. The likelihood of working full-time increased even more, by over 400%. Working by other household members stayed relatively constant.

A majority (56%) of our total panel reported working at either 12 or 24 months after giving birth; 23% reported working at both those times. Of the 310 women who remained in the study panel for 36 months, over two thirds (69%) reported working at some time during follow-up and 20% were working at all three follow-up waves.

Table 1 also shows trends in combinations of welfare and work in the household. A small percentage of the women combined welfare with working; this percentage was lowest in late pregnancy (8%) and ranged from 11% to 15% in the three years following the birth. A larger minority of the women were neither working nor on AFDC at any given time; the percentage in this combination increased somewhat over time, from

TABLE 1. Welfare Participation, Work, Fertility, and Well-Being Over Time

Predictors	Time relative to birth			
	Late pregnancy (n = 435)	12 M (n = 435)	24 M (n = 435)	36 M (n = 310)
Respondent on AFDC[a] (%)	80.0[c]	65.9	44.7	46.4
Someone in household working (%)	59.8	66.6	65.2	76.1
Respondent working (%)				
Part time	6.7	14.0	17.6	14.6
Full time	5.8	12.3	28.3	29.2
Total	12.5	26.3	45.9	43.8
Other household member working (%)	55.2	56.0	59.4	54.1
Welfare & work combination (%)				
AFDC[a] & not working	72.5	54.5	29.6	30.9
AFDC[a] & working	7.5	11.4	15.1	12.9
Not working & no AFDC[a]	15.0	19.2	24.5	22.7
Working & no AFDC[a]	5.0	14.9	30.8	33.5
No AFDC[a] & none in household working (%)	2.5	2.6	5.1	4.2
Pregnancy/birth[b] (%)	100.0	12.0	32.5	28.7
Difficult life circumstances (DLC) (M)	3.8	3.9	3.4	2.5
Depression (CES-D) (M)	17.0	14.3	13.1	13.3

[a]TANF, after July 1997
[b]Pregnant or gave birth in last 12M, may overlap across time periods
[c]On AFDC during pregnancy or within 6M of birth

15% during late pregnancy to over 20% after two years. Most of this group had other household members working but a very small percentage of the sample, increasing over time from 2% to about 4%, had no discernable source of support in the household. At any given time most of the women (60%-78%) were either on welfare or working, but not both. Over time, the percentage only working increased as the percentage only on welfare declined.

Figure 1 shows the trends in working part or full time across the three-year period by whether the women initially participated in AFDC. Compared with non-welfare participants, women initially on AFDC were less likely to work during pregnancy and at 12 months, but after the first year the pattern reversed. At 24 and 36 months mothers who had initially been welfare recipients were more likely to be employed than mothers who had not. In fact, women who initially depended on welfare were more likely to have participated in the labor force at some time during the study than those who had not, at both 24 months (58% vs. 51%) and 36 months (72% vs. 58%) after giving birth. These results suggest that taking welfare around the time of birth not only did not in-

FIGURE 1. Full-Time, Part-Time Work by Initial AFDC Status Over Time

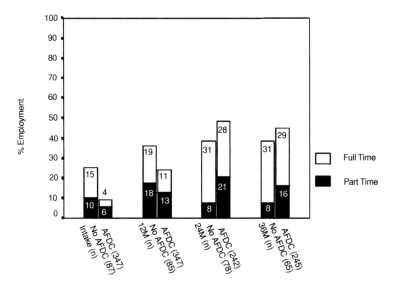

Initial AFDC Status, by Month

hibit a mother's later employment, but may have even facilitated it. However, initial AFDC participation was associated with a lower likelihood of working full time.

All the women in our study panel were pregnant at intake. After that, the likelihood at any given wave of a participant again being pregnant or having recently given birth increased from 12% in the first year to 29% in the third. Overall, 35% of the women had a repeat pregnancy within the first two years, and 44% of those who remained in the panel for 36 months had a pregnancy during that period. The likelihood of repeat pregnancy was not related to initial welfare status.

Maternal well-being tended to increase as the babies grew older. During pregnancy and at 12 months, the average respondent reported about four difficult life circumstances in her life; by 36 months, the number of difficulties had declined to 2.5. The mean CES-D score of 17 (symptom days per week) for the sample during late pregnancy was above the cutoff suggested for referral to outpatient treatment; however, the scores decreased over time to an average of 13 at 36 months.

Factors Influencing Employment

For our second and third research goals we used logistic- and linear-regression software (Hedeker & Gibbons, 1996a, 1996b) to perform multi-level (random effects) regression with time-dependent variables nested within individuals. These analytic techniques permit us to include in the models respondents who have only three waves of data (through 24 months), as well as those interviewed in all four waves (through 36 months). In all models, to accommodate clustering within individuals we tested both the intercept and the time coefficient as random effects.

The second research goal was to model a woman's work participation over this period on the basis of personal and household characteristics, initial welfare participation and fertility over time. Multi-level logistic regression was used to model employment status at 12, 24 and 36 months (Hedeker & Gibbons, 1996a). We modeled *working at all* separately from *full-time employment*. Non-time-varying predictors in these models were mother's ethnicity, age, parity, education, household employment experience, birth cohort and initial welfare participation.

In using a respondent's own work experience to predict her later employment status there is a danger of endogeneity; that is, coefficients in a model can be biased if unmeasured variables affect both the predictor and the outcome (Allison, 1999). Realizing this, but nonetheless wishing to use this important aspect of human capital as a predictor, we tested three alternate versions of each model employing different indicators of work experience that would not share the same sources of bias. The first used only employment of another household member in the last 12 months to represent the work experience. The second added recent employment on the part of the respondent to recent employment of another household member. The third added whether the respondent had ever worked for six months to recent work experience of other household member(s). Time and fertility were nested within individuals in all the models. In addition to main effects, we tested for interactions among ethnicity, initial welfare participation and time.

Models for work. Table 2 summarizes a model that describes the impact of different predictors on whether a respondent was working at any given time. In these models both the intercept and the time coefficient were treated as random effects; that is, the two coefficients were permitted to vary across individuals. Testing for two- and three-way interactions among ethnicity, initial AFDC status and time, we found that initial AFDC status interacted separately with race

TABLE 2. Multi-Level Logistic Regression Models for Predicting Work Over Time[a]

Predictors	Models for work					
	1		2		3	
	OR[b]	p[c]	OR[b]	p[c]	OR[b]	p[c]
Teen	.81	n.s.	.90	n.s.	1.54	n.s.
H.S. or G.E.D.	6.30	<.01	4.06	<.01	3.86	<.01
Multiparous	.90	n.s.	.91	n.s.	.97	n.s.
Birth cohort	1.58	n.s.	1.48	n.s.	1.68	n.s.
Initial AFDC	.25	<.10	.36	n.s.	.20	<.05
Other worked in last 12M	2.18	<.05	4.26	<.01	1.86	<.10
R worked in last 12M			9.02	<.01		
R had 6M work experience					8.41	<.01
Repeat pregnancy	.38	<.01	.42	<.01	.41	<.01
Af. Am/No AFDC[d]	6.49	<.01	5.93	<.01	4.85	<.01
Time/No AFDC[d]	1.00	n.s.	1.00	n.s.	1.00	n.s.
Af. Am/ AFDC[d]	1.22	n.s.	1.00	n.s.	1.22	n.s.
Time/ AFDC[d]	1.08	<.05	1.08	<.05	1.08	<.05

[a] Models with two random effects: intercept and time
[b] Odds ratio
[c] Two-tailed
[d] Effects contingent on initial AFDC status

and with time (p < .05, not shown). Models 1, 2 and 3 are three versions of the model for work. In addition to the main effects of other predictors, they present the interaction of initial AFDC status with ethnicity and time by making the effect of these contingent on initial AFDC status. Models 1, 2 and 3 differ in that they incorporate different indicators of household work experience as predictors for working. These models show that a woman was more likely to work after the birth of her baby if she had a high school degree or equivalent and if she and/or another household member had prior work experience. Her likelihood of working was depressed by a repeat pregnancy, but otherwise increased as her baby grew older.

In these multi-level models initial welfare participation was associated with a somewhat decreased likelihood of working (significantly so in two of the three equations), but the actual effect of welfare participation depended on a combination of ethnicity and baby's age. Among women initially on AFDC, African Americans and Mexican Americans were equally likely to work and their work participation increased as their babies grew older. This increasing trend in working over the three-year period among mothers initially on welfare is evident in Figure 1. Among those not initially on AFDC, their likelihood of working did not vary with the age of their babies, but African American mothers were more likely to work than their Mexican American peers. Age, parity and birth cohort were not related to a woman's likelihood of working.

Models for full time work. Table 3 summarizes the logistic models for predicting full-time employment. These models were estimated as random intercept (only) models, because there was no significant variation associated with the random effect of time. There were no interaction effects among ethnicity, initial welfare participation and time on the likelihood of working full-time, so we present only main effect models. Models 1, 2 and 3 show that the likelihood of full-time employment was enhanced by a high school education and time since birth, and inhibited by repeat pregnancy. Multiparous women and women initially on AFDC were somewhat less likely to work full-time (in two of three equations for each). In Model 2, recent work experience on her own part and on the part of another household member independently increased a woman's likelihood of working full-time after having a baby. In Model 3, the likelihood of full-time work was higher for women who had at least six months of work experience. These results suggest that a woman's own employment experience may have been a more important influence than the employment experience of other household members on her likelihood of working full-time.

Robustness of the employment models. Using initial AFDC status and repeat pregnancy as predictors in models for predicting work might result in biased coefficients if welfare, work and pregnancy were responses to common unmeasured conditions. To evaluate this possibility, we reestimated the models for employment after eliminating both initial AFDC and repeat pregnancy as predictors. Removing these covariates from the models had virtually no effect on the coefficients for other predictors of working or working full-time. The models also yielded similar findings for three different measures of household work experience. The consistent results across different model specifications encourage cautious confidence in the robustness of our models for employment among low-income inner city mothers of young children.

Work and Well-Being

The third research goal was to consider the impact of employment and other predictors on maternal well-being. We were particularly interested in determining the effect of working on different aspects of

TABLE 3. Multi-Level Logistic Regression Models for Predicting Full-Time Work Over Time[a]

Predictors	Models for full-time work					
	1		2		3	
	OR[b]	p[c]	OR[b]	p[c]	OR[b]	p[c]
African American	1.03	n.s.	.90	n.s.	.95	n.s.
Teen	.66	n.s.	.79	n.s.	1.20	n.s.
H.S. or G.E.D.	5.64	<.01	3.97	<.01	3.86	<.01
Multiparous	.53	<.10	.54	<.10	.64	n.s.
Birth cohort	1.43	n.s.	1.32	n.s.	1.45	n.s.
Initial AFDC	.52	<.10	.45	n.s.	.76	<.05
Other worked in last 12M	1.20	n.s.	2.32	<.05	1.04	n.s.
R worked in last 12M			7.03	<.01		
R had 6M work experience					7.24	<.01
Time (Baby's age)	1.07	<.01	1.07	<.01	1.07	<.01
Repeat pregnancy	.44	<.01	.47	<.01	.44	<.01

[a] Random intercept models
[b] Odds ratio.
[c] Two-tailed

well-being after controlling for factors that might influence the likelihood of working. We used multi-level linear regression (Hedeker & Gibbons, 1996b) to model the two aspects of well-being–difficult life circumstances and depression–over time (from 12 through 36 months). In these models we started with the same predictors for employment as in the main effect models, then added current employment status (either working or working full-time) to time and fertility as a time-varying factor nested within individuals.

Models for difficult life circumstances. Table 4 summarizes the models for predicting difficult life circumstances in the three years after the baby was born. Models 1, 2 and 3 predict this indicator of negative well-being as a function of personal characteristics, birth cohort, household work experience, time, repeat pregnancy and employment. Women with previous children and those initially participating in AFDC experienced a larger number of difficult life circumstances but, in general, the number of life circumstances declined over time as the babies grew older. Difficult life circumstances were unrelated to ethnicity, age, education, birth cohort, work experience on the part of the woman or other household members, or repeat pregnancy. Controlling for these prior predictors, adding working per se to the models did not influence the number of difficult life circumstances (these equations not shown). However, when other predictors

TABLE 4. Multi-Level Linear Regression Models for Predicting Difficult Life Circumstances (DLC)[a]

Predictors	Models for DLC					
	1		2		3	
	b	p[b]	b	p[b]	b	p[b]
Intercept	3.32	<.01	3.34	<.01	3.23	<.01
African American	.03	n.s.	−.02	n.s.	−.04	n.s.
Teen	−.19	n.s.	−.19	n.s.	−.14	n.s.
H.S. or G.E.D.	−.33	n.s.	−.33	n.s.	−.37	n.s.
Multiparous	.57	<.05	.57	<.05	.58	<.05
Birth cohort	.05	n.s.	.05	n.s.	.05	n.s.
Initial AFDC	.88	<.01	.87	<.01	.86	<.01
Other worked in last 12M	.06	n.s.	.05	n.s.	.05	n.s.
R worked in last 12M			−.03	n.s.		
R had 6M work experience					.18	n.s.
Time (Baby's age)	−.01	<.05	−.01	<.05	−.01	<.05
Repeat pregnancy	−.25	n.s.	−.25	n.s.	−.24	n.s.
Full time work	−.45	<.05	−.45	<.05	−.46	<.05

[a] Models with two random effects: intercept and time
[b] Two-tailed

were controlled, working full-time did reduce the reported number of difficult life circumstances by .45-.46, or about half an event.

Models for depression. Table 5 summarizes the models for predicting CES-D scores over time. Models 1, 2 and 3 show that women with a high school education and at least six months of work experience reported less frequent depressive symptoms. Initial AFDC participation and repeated pregnancy were associated with elevated CES-D scores. Controlling for all these factors, depressive symptoms tended to decrease as the babies aged. Ethnicity, age, parity, birth cohort and recent work experience on the part of the mother or other household members were not related to depression. When we added employment status to these models, neither working at all nor working full-time had any effect on depression scores.

DISCUSSION

A substantial body of research has documented the contribution of human capital investments, particularly high school education and

TABLE 5. Multi-Level Linear Regression Models for Predicting Depression (CES-D)[a]

| Predictors | Models for CES-D | | | | | |
| | 1 | | 2 | | 3 | |
	b	p[b]	b	p[b]	b	p[b]
Intercept	14.08	<.01	14.69	<.01	15.08	<.01
African American	−1.29	n.s.	−1.21	n.s.	−1.16	n.s.
Teen	.84	n.s.	.76	n.s.	.16	n.s.
H.S. or G.E.D.	−2.96	<.01	−2.67	<.01	−2.58	<.01
Multiparous	1.21	n.s.	1.21	n.s.	1.02	n.s.
Birth cohort	.02	n.s.	.06	n.s.	.05	n.s.
Initial AFDC	3.01	<.01	2.77	<.05	3.19	<.01
Other worked in last 12 months	−.62	n.s.	−1.01	n.s.	−.46	n.s.
R worked in last 12 months			−1.53	n.s.		
R had 6 months work experience					−2.09	<.05
Time (Baby's age)	−.06	<.01	−.06	<.01	−.06	<.01
Repeat pregnancy	1.43	<.05	1.41	<.05	1.49	<.05

[a] Random intercept models
[b] Two-tailed

work experience, on the employability of poor, inner-city women. These results have already been shown for a national sample of AFDC recipients in the mid-1980s (Harris, 1993, 1996); poor, single mothers in urban Massachusetts from 1992 to 1995 (Brooks & Buckner, 1996); various national longitudinal surveys and multi-site evaluations of welfare-to-work strategies in the late pre-TANF period (Kalil et al., 1998; Martinson, 2000); and non-Hispanic TANF recipients in urban Michigan (Danziger et al., 2000) and African American, white and Hispanic TANF recipients in Illinois (IDHS, 2000b) during the early TANF period. Our research, bridging the late pre-TANF and early-TANF periods and focusing on African American and Mexican American women in Chicago, further supports the importance of these aspects of human capital. Extending the conceptualization of work experience to include the recent work experience of other household members, we found others' experience to facilitate working at least part-time, though there was a weaker effect on full-time work. However, our findings do not support the expectation, based upon the same body of research, that teen mothers, multiparous women, and those who receive welfare benefits when their children are infants, are less likely to participate in the labor force.

There is some evidence that having more than one child may depress a woman's odds of working full-time, but it does not affect her overall likelihood of working.

The effect of initial welfare participation on employment seems in particular to be much more complex than is evident in earlier research, interacting with both ethnicity and the age of the baby. Among women on welfare around the time of birth, there was an increasing tendency to enter the labor force as the baby grew older. Rather than inhibiting working, by allowing a woman to concentrate on parenting responsibilities at this critical time in the family life cycle, the initial welfare participation may actually have facilitated later employment activity. However, this encouraging effect did not extend to working full-time.

The influence of the family life cycle on maternal employment has been established. One contribution of our research is documentation of the specific importance of timing and family life events in the welfare-to-work process. Around the birth of a child small increments in time make a big difference in a woman's ability to work, and repeat pregnancies depress labor force participation by more than half. These findings suggest that modification of TANF might productively incorporate reproductive health care to help a woman in the welfare-to-work process avoid unintended pregnancy.

Data collection for our study bridged two welfare policy periods–JOBS and early TANF. Given the similar Illinois policies in these periods perhaps it is not surprising that we found no effects of birth cohort on work or well-being outcomes. Research literature spanning at least two decades of welfare policies has documented substantial work activity on the part of welfare recipients. Welfare reforms have had more effect on welfare participation than on labor force involvement. A major effect on employment rates is the economic environment, which was strong during our study period. One must be cautious in interpreting effects of welfare reforms in the context of an expanding economy. What will happen to these women when the economy slows?

Given the incentives in Illinois to combine welfare with work to enhance family income, we expected a woman's employment to ameliorate difficult circumstances in her life. However, controlling for factors predictive of working, working alone had no relation to number of difficult circumstances reported. Only full-time work predicted difficult life circumstances; respondents reported about .5 fewer difficulties during periods of full-time employment. The causal order for this association is not clear. We found no evidence for our tentative expectations that work–either full- or part-time–would contribute to our respondents' psychological well-being in the form of reduced depression. This may be because the jobs available to them are neither challenging or interesting, nor likely to lead to self-sufficiency.

Our research has documented the family life cycle as a strong influence on maternal well-being. The well-being of mothers increased–whether viewed as rates of difficult life circumstances or of depression–as their babies grew older. To understand influences on work and well-being, evaluations of welfare policy must take into account the family life cycle, focusing on much smaller increments of time around the birth of a child.

REFERENCES

Allison, P. (1999). *Multiple regression.* Thousand Oaks, CA: Pine Forge Press.

Aneshensel, C. S., Frerichs, R. R., & Clark, V. A. (1981). Family roles and sex differences in depression. *Journal of Health and Social Behavior, 22,* 379-393.

Annie E. Casey Foundation (1999). *Kids count data book: State profiles of child well-being.* Baltimore: Annie E. Casey Foundation.

Barnard, K. (1989). *NCAST difficult life circumstances manual.* Seattle, WA: NCAST Publications, University of Washington, School of Nursing.

Becker, G. S. (1993). *Human capital: A theoretical & empirical analysis with special reference to education* (3rd Ed). Chicago: University of Chicago Press.

Bourdieu, P. (1986). The forms of capital. In J. G. Richardson (Ed.), *Handbook of theory and research for the sociology of education* (pp. 241-258). New York: Greenwood Press.

Boyd, C., Norr, K., & Nacion, K. (2001). Promoting infant health through home visiting by a nurse community worker team. *Journal of Public Health Nursing* (In press).

Boyd, J. M., Weissman, M. M., Thompson, D., & Myers, J. K. (1982). Screening for depression in a community sample. *Archives of General Psychiatry, 19,* 1195-1200.

Brooks, M., & Buckner, J. (1996). Work and welfare: Job histories, barriers to employment, and predictors of work among low-income single mothers. *American Journal of Orthopsychiatry, 66* (4), 526-537.

Budig, M., & England, P. (2001). The wage penalty for motherhood. *American Sociological Review, 66,* 204-225.

Burtless, G. (1997). Welfare recipients' job skills and employment prospects. In R. E. Behrman (Ed.), *The future of children* (pp. 39-51). Los Altos, CA: The Center for the Future of Children, The Davis and Lucile Packard Foundation.

Carlson, V., & Theodore, N. (1997). Employment availability for entry-level workers: An examination of the spatial mismatch hypothesis in Chicago. *Urban Geography, March.*

Cho, Y. I. (1999). *The effects of adult roles on drinking among women in the United States.* Unpublished doctoral dissertation, University of Illinois at Chicago, Chicago.

Danziger, S., Corcoran, M., Danziger, S., Heflin, C., Kalil, A., Levine, J., Rosen, D., Seefeldt, K., Siefert, K., & Tolman, R. (2000). *Barriers to the employment of welfare recipients.* Michigan: University of Michigan, Poverty Research & Training Center.

Ellwood, D. (1988). *Poor support: Poverty in the American family.* New York: Basic Books.

Freedman, S., Friedlander, D., Hamilton, G., Rock, J., Mitchell, M., Nudelman, J., Schweder, A., & Storto, L. (2000). *National evaluation of welfare-to-work strategies. Evaluating alternative welfare-to-work approaches: Two-year impacts for eleven programs.* Washington, DC: U.S. Department of Health and Human Services, Administration for Children and Families, Office of the Assistant Secretary for Planning and Evaluation; and U.S. Department of Education, Office of the Under Secretary and Office of Vocational and Adult Education.

Harris, K. M. (1993). Work and welfare among single mothers in poverty. *American Journal of Sociology, 99,* 317-352.

Harris, K. M. (1996). Life after welfare: Women, work, and repeat dependency. *American Sociological Review, 61,* 407-426.

Hedeker, D., & Gibbons, R. D. (1996a). MIXOR: A computer program for mixed-effects ordinal regression analysis. *Computer Methods and Programs in Biomedicine, 49,* 157-176.

Hedeker, D., & Gibbons, R. D. (1996b). MIXREG: A computer program for mixed-effects regression analysis with autocorrelated errors. *Computer Methods and Programs in Biomedicine, 49,* 229-252.

Henle, T., & Ali, E. (1996). Welfare reform and child care. In Illinois Job Gap Project (Ed.), *The welfare reform debate: Critical policy issues* (pp. 17-26). Illinois: Illinois Job Gap Project.

Henle, T., & Kinsella, A. (1996). Welfare reform and transportation to work. In Illinois Job Gap Project (Ed.), *The welfare reform debate: Critical policy issues* (pp. 27-40). Illinois: Illinois Job Gap Project.

Holzer, H. (1996). *What employers want: Job prospects for less-educated workers.* New York: Russell Sage Foundation.

Illinois Department of Human Services (2000a). *Child care and subsidy use in Illinois.* Springfield, IL: Illinois Department of Human Services.

Illinois Department of Human Services (2000b). *Illinois study of former TANF clients: Final report.* Springfield, IL: Illinois Department of Human Services.

Illinois Department of Public Aid (1995). *Report to the General Assembly: Child care programs.* Springfield, IL: Illinois Department of Public Aid.

Illinois Department of Public Aid (1997). *State of Illinois: Plan for temporary assistance for needy families.* Springfield, IL: Illinois Department of Public Aid.

Joseph, L. (1999). Introduction. In L. Joseph (Ed.), *Families, poverty, and welfare reform* (pp. 1-34). Champaign, IL: University of Illinois Press.

Kalil, A., Corcoran, M. E., Danziger, S. K., Tolman, R., Seefeldt, K. S., Rosen, D., & Nam, Y. (1998). *Getting jobs, keeping jobs, and earning a living wage: Can welfare reform work?* Michigan: University of Michigan, Institute for Research on Poverty, Discussion Paper (No. 1170-98).

Leathers, S. J., Kelley, M. A., & Richman, J. A. (1997). Postpartum depressive symptomatology in new mothers and fathers: Parenting, work, and support. *The Journal of Nervous and Mental Disease, 185,* 129-139.

Lewis, D., George, C., & Puntenney, D. (1999). Welfare reform effects in Illinois. In L. Joseph (Ed.), *Families, poverty, and welfare reform* (pp. 99-138). Champaign, IL: University of Illinois Press.

Logsdon, M. C., McBride, A. B., & Birkimer, J. C. (1994). Social support and postpartum depression. *Research in Nursing & Health, 17,* 449-457.

Martinson, K. (2000). *The national evaluation of welfare-to-work strategies: The experience of welfare recipients who find jobs.* Washington, DC: U.S. Department of Health and Human Services, Administration for Children and Families, Office of the Assistant Secretary for Planning and Evaluation; and U.S. Department of Education, Office of the Under Secretary and Office of Vocational and Adult Education.

Myers, J. K., & Weissman, M. M. (1980). Use of a self-report symptom scale to detect depression in a community sample. *American Journal of Psychiatry, 137,* 1081-1084.

Orme, J. G., Reis, J., & Herz, E. J. (1986). Factorial and discriminant validity of the Center for Epidemiologic Studies Depression (CES-D) scale. *Journal of Clinical Psychology, 42,* 28-33.

Ortiz, V., & Fennelly, K. (1988). Early childbearing and employment among young Mexican origin, black, and white women. *Social Science Quarterly, 69,* 987-995.

Pavetti, L. (1996). *How much more can they work? A comparison of the work experiences of welfare recipients and non-recipients.* Washington, DC: Urban Institute.

Radloff, L. S. (1977). The CES-D Scale: A self-report depression scale for research in the general population. *Applied Psychological Measurement, 1,* 385-401.

Radloff, L. S., & Locke, B. Z. (1986). The community mental health assessment survey and the CES-D scale. In M. M. Weissman, J. K. Myers, & C. E. Ross (Eds.), *Community surveys of psychiatric disorders* (pp. 177-189). New Brunswick: Rutgers University Press.

Roberts, R. E., & Vernon, S. W. (1983). The Center for Epidemiologic Studies Depression scale: Its use in a community sample. *American Journal of Psychiatry, 140,* 41-46.

Santor, D. A., Zuroff, D. C., Ramsay, J. O., Cervantes, P., & Palacios, J. (1995). Examining the scale discriminability in the BDI and CES-D as a function of depressive severity. *Psychological Assessment, 7,* 131-139.

Spalter-Roth, R., Burr, B., Hartmann, H., & Shaw, L. (1995). *Welfare that works: The working lives of AFDC recipients.* Washington, DC: Institute for Women's Policy Research.

Thoits, P. A. (1991). On merging identity theory and stress research. *Social Psychology Quarterly, 54,* 101-112.

U.S. Census (1990). *Annual demographic survey.* [On line]. Available: http://ferret.bls.census.gov/macro/031996/pov/1_000.htm.

U.S. Department of Health and Human Services (USDHHS) (1996). *State welfare demonstrations.* [On line]. Available: http://www.os.dhhs.gov/news/press/1996pres/961007b.html.

Waite, L. J., Haggstrom, G. W., & Kanouse. D. E. (1985). Changes in the employment activities of new parents. *American Sociological Review, 50*, 263-72.

Weissman, M. M., Sholomskas, D., Pottenger, M., Prusoff, B. A., & Locke, B. Z. (1977). Assessing depressive symptoms in five psychiatric populations: A validation study. *American Journal of Epidemiology, 106*, 203-214.

How Do Maternal Risk Factors
Affect Children in Low-Income Families?
Further Evidence
of Two-Generational Implications

Elizabeth C. Hair
Sharon M. McGroder
Martha J. Zaslow
Surjeet K. Ahluwalia
Kristin A. Moore

Child Trends

Address correspondence to: Elizabeth Hair, Child Trends, 4301 Connecticut Avenue, NW, Suite 100, Washington, DC 20008 (E-mail: ehair@childtrends.org).

The authors gratefully acknowledge discussions with Peggy Hamburg (former Assistant Secretary for Planning and Evaluation), Ann Segal, Martha Moorehouse, and Audrey Mirsky-Ashby (of ASPE, DHHS) that led to the identification of low literacy and maternal depressive symptoms as particularly important potential barriers in families receiving welfare. This paper uses data from the JOBS Observational Study, as well as from the Child Outcomes Study of the National Evaluation of Welfare-to-Work Strategies. The authors thank their co-investigators in the JOBS Observational Study for their input at many levels (from conceptualizing of the observational study through data collection and coding), including (in alphabetical order) Jeanne De Temple, Byron Egeland, Carolyn Eldred, Robert Granger, Donna Morrison, John Ogawa, Catherine Snow, Patton Tabors, and Nancy Weinfeld. The JOBS Observational Study is funded by the Foundation for Child Development, the William T. Grant Foundation, the George Gund Foundation, with funds for pretest work also provided by the U.S. Department of Health and Human Services.

This research would not have been possible without the permission and financial support of officials from the Secretary's Office of Planning and Evaluation of the U.S. Department of Health and Human Services, which funded the Manpower Demonstration Research Corporation (MDRC) to direct the National Evaluation of Welfare-to-Work strategies and Child Trends to conduct the Child Outcomes Study (contract #HHS-100-89-0030).

[Haworth co-indexing entry note]: "How Do Maternal Risk Factors Affect Children in Low-Income Families? Further Evidence of Two-Generational Implications." Hair, Elizabeth C. et al. Co-published simultaneously in *Journal of Prevention & Intervention in the Community* (The Haworth Press, Inc.) Vol. 23, No. 1/2, 2002, pp. 65-94; and: *The Transition from Welfare to Work: Processes, Challenges, and Outcomes* (ed: Sharon Telleen, and Judith V. Sayad) The Haworth Press, Inc., 2002, pp. 65-94. Single or multiple copies of this article are available for a fee from The Haworth Document Delivery Service [1-800-HAWORTH, 9:00 a.m. - 5:00 p.m. (EST). E-mail address: getinfo@haworthpressinc.com].

SUMMARY. This longitudinal study examines the role of depressive symptoms and low literacy among mothers receiving welfare in predicting outcomes for both parents and children (mothers' psychological and employment-related outcomes and children's development across multiple domains). For African-American single mothers (n = 351), depressive symptoms in mothers are an important predictor of their later psychological well-being, while maternal literacy affects both their participation in welfare-to-work activities and later employment. An analysis of the academic functioning of children found a main effect for maternal literacy. Maternal literacy also significantly interacted with maternal depression. The children of mothers with a greater number of depressive symptoms had less favorable cognitive achievement outcomes when their mothers also had low literacy. Structural equation models indicate that parenting behavior mediates the relationship between depressive symptoms, literacy and later child outcomes. Among mothers with low literacy the pathways linking depressive symptoms, parenting, and child outcomes are stronger. *[Article copies available for a fee from The Haworth Document Delivery Service: 1-800-HAWORTH. E-mail address: <getinfo@haworthpressinc.com> Website: <http://www.HaworthPress.com> © 2002 by The Haworth Press, Inc. All rights reserved.]*

KEYWORDS. Low-income women, depression, literacy, child outcomes, TANF

The earliest welfare policies in the United States were designed as a safety net for the children of widows. In the decades that followed, as never-married mothers increasingly comprised the welfare caseload and as societal attitudes toward maternal employment became more favorable, welfare polices focused increasingly on facilitating maternal employment as the means for improving low-income families' economic circumstances. The most recent reform of the welfare system, the Personal Responsibility and Work Opportunity Reconciliation Act of 1996, replaced the 60-year-old entitlement to a federal safety net known as Aid to Families with Dependent Children (AFDC) with Temporary Assistance to Needy Families (TANF), a program of time-limited assistance that required employment for mothers with children as young as 12 months (and younger at state option).

Welfare caseloads dropped precipitously in the 1990s, with a 50% decrease in the number of families receiving TANF since the signing of the welfare law in August, 1996 (Administration for Children and Families, 2000). In addition to welfare policies' increased emphasis on work, scholars and policy analysts also credit a booming economy and the expansion of anti-poverty programs that reward work, such as the federal Earned Income Tax Credit, for much of this decline (Moffitt, 1999).

With such beneficial trends in policy and the economy, one result of this convergence of work incentive policies may be that those long-term recipients who remain on the caseloads are those who face multiple or particularly debilitating barriers to employment (Brooks & Buckner, 1996; Danziger et al., 1999; Olson & Pavetti, 1996; Seefeldt, 2001). At the same time, while identifying and addressing such barriers are imperative for moving welfare recipients into employment, the motivating force behind welfare policy in this country has always been the well-being of the children in these families, and it remains important not to lose sight of this.

Factors characterized as "barriers" to employment in the welfare literature often also emerge in the developmental literature as risk factors in children's development. One such barrier is recipients' limited "human capital," including low basic skills and literacy, as well as limited educational attainment. Researchers have documented lower rates of employment for low-income mothers with low basic skills (Olson & Pavetti, 1996; Zaslow, McGroder, Cave, & Mariner, 1999) and for those without a high school diploma or GED (Brooks & Buckner, 1996; Danziger et al., 1999; McGroder, Papillo, & Zaslow, 2001), and higher rates of employment for low-income mothers with some post-secondary training or schooling (McGroder et al., 2001). Just as limited human capital is a primary barrier to maternal employment (Olson & Pavetti, 1996), it is a key predictor of children's later educational attainment (Haveman & Wolfe, 1995). Mothers' parenting behavior may play a role in these children's academic outcomes; studies have shown less educated mothers to be less responsive (McLeod & Shanahan, 1993) and to provide a less stimulating home environment (Goodman & Brumley, 1990; McGroder, 2000) than their more highly educated counterparts.

Maternal depression also can be seen to be both a barrier to employment and a risk factor for children. Mental health problems generally are among the most prevalent barriers to employment faced by individuals receiving welfare (Danziger, Kalil, & Anderson, 2000; Lennon, Blome, & English, 2001). Danziger and colleagues found that welfare recipients who meet the diagnostic criteria for a major depressive disorder were less likely than non-depressed recipients to be working at least

20 hours per week (Danziger et al., 1999). Maternal depression also places children at risk for less optimal developmental outcomes, with less responsive or hostile and/or harsh parenting serving as likely conduits (Goodman & Brumley, 1990; McGroder, 2000; McLoyd, 1990).

An earlier study of a sample of families with a history of prior welfare receipt suggested that low maternal literacy and high maternal depressive symptoms may have "two-generational" implications for the employment outcomes of mothers and the developmental outcomes of their children (Zaslow, Hair, Dion, Ahluwalia, & Sargent, 2001). The initial study found that mothers who had applied for or were receiving welfare and who had low levels of baseline literacy were less likely to be employed two years later, though relatively numerous depressive symptoms did not predict subsequent employment. Low maternal literacy served as a risk factor for 5- to 7-year-olds' cognitive school readiness but not for their behavioral outcomes, whereas numerous maternal depressive symptoms served as a risk factor for children's behavioral but not cognitive outcomes. Internalizing behaviors were greatest for children whose mothers had both low literacy and numerous depressive symptoms. As hypothesized, observational measures of supportive and cognitively stimulating parenting mediated the relationship between these maternal risk factors measured early on and the children's subsequent developmental outcomes, with the effects of maternal depressive symptoms on parenting strongest for mothers with low literacy. That is, depressive symptoms more strongly predicted measures of parenting–and, consequently, more strongly affected child outcomes–in the presence of low literacy than in the presence of higher literacy. It appears that higher literacy acts as a buffer against the unfavorable patterns of parenting and child outcomes often found to be associated with maternal depression.

The present study replicates and extends the findings of Zaslow et al. (2001), and seeks to gain a better understanding of the long-term implications of maternal depressive symptoms and low literacy by examining mothers' employment and children's behavioral and educational outcomes five years later. This study examines a broader set of employment-related outcomes–including participation in welfare-to-work activities, employment at the five-year follow-up, and any employment over the five-year period–and examines mothers' recurrent depressive symptoms over this period in light of earlier levels of maternal literacy and depressive symptoms. It also looks beyond children's academic school readiness at school entry to children's achievement and engagement in school three years later, when children were between about 8 and 10 years old. We hypothesize that the relation between maternal risk factors and children's subsequent outcomes will endure through the elementary school years, with children whose mothers had low literacy and reported greater depressive symptoms five years earlier faring more poorly than children whose mothers had none or only one of these risks. We again examine the role played by observational measures of parenting, and hypothesize that (1) parenting will continue to mediate the relation between antecedent maternal risks and subsequent child outcomes, and (2) higher literacy will continue to buffer the negative effects of depressive symptoms on parenting.

METHOD

Design

Data for the present set of analyses come from the Observational Study that follows participants in the Job Opportunities and Basic Skills Training Program (JOBS). JOBS is the name given to the set of welfare-to-work programs put in place nationally under the Family Support Act of 1988. The JOBS Observational Study is a longitudinal study focusing on parenting in a sample of mothers who had applied for or were receiving welfare. The Observational Study is embedded in a larger evaluation study, the Child Outcomes Study of the National Evaluation of Welfare-to-Work Strategies (NEWWS). The larger Child Outcomes Study is examining the impacts on children of their mothers' assignment to participate in the JOBS Program (see McGroder, Zaslow, Moore, & LeMenestrel, 2000). In the three NEWWS sites selected for the Child Outcomes Study (Atlanta, Georgia; Riverside, California; Grand Rapids, Michigan), the mothers were randomly assigned to a control group (eligible for all benefits associated with AFDC, but free of the requirement to participate in welfare-to-work activities) or to one of two program groups in which mothers were eligible for AFDC, but for whom participation in a JOBS welfare-to-work program was mandatory. One program emphasized a rapid transition to employment, known as labor force attachment, while the other focused first on building human capital through basic education and training, known as human capital development. In each family one child became the focus for observation and assessment. Focal children in the Child Outcomes Study ranged from three to five years of age at baseline.

The Observational Study was carried out in a sub-sample of the Child Outcomes Study from the Atlanta, Georgia site. Families were enrolled in the Observational Study from among the 790 families who were part of the Descriptive Study (see Moore, Zaslow, Coiro, Miller, & Magenheim, 1995). Only families from the control group and the human capital development program group were enrolled. The sample was also limited to families in which the focal child was between three and four years of age at baseline because the observational procedures for examining the mother-child interactions were only appropriate for this age range

Of those invited to participate, 372 families (83 percent) completed Wave 1 of the study. Comparing baseline characteristics of those eligible families who did participate with those who did not, there was no evidence of a systematic difference. There was also no systematic difference between those in the control group and those in the program group.

Observational Study families provided information at six time points: baseline (time of enrollment in the study, with data collected prior to random assignment); the Descriptive Study (about three months after baseline); Wave 1 of the Observational Study (about five months after baseline); the two-year follow-up of the larger evaluation; Wave 2 of the Observational Study (about four-and-a-half years after baseline); and the five-year follow-up of the larger Child Outcomes Study. The present set of analyses focuses on data from four of the six points of data collection available for the Observational Study sample: (1) baseline (T1); (2) the Descriptive Study (T2); (3) Wave 1 of the Observational Study (T3); and (4) data from the five-year follow-up (T4).

Sample

For purposes of the present set of analyses, we focus on 351 of the 372 families who completed the procedures of Wave 1 of the Observational Study. Table 1 shows baseline characteristics of these 351 families. Mothers averaged 29 years of age at baseline and children averaged 49.2 months. Almost three quarters of the mothers had never been married. The mothers averaged 21.5 years at the birth of the first child. The majority of the mothers had only one or two children. Nearly two thirds of the mothers had completed high school or a GED. Two thirds of the mothers had worked full-time for six months or more for the same employer, as of baseline, though nearly 80 percent had had no earnings in the year prior to baseline. Almost 36 percent had been in a family that received AFDC during their childhood. About two in ten of the mothers

TABLE 1. Selected Baseline Characteristics of Wave 1 JOBS Observational Study Sample *(n* = 351)

Characteristics	Mean	Percent
Demographic Characteristics		
Age of Focal Child (months)	49.2	
Marital Status Never Married Ever Married		72.1 28.0
Maternal age (years)	29.3	
Age at first birth (years)	21.5	
Number of Children One child Two children Three or more children		25.1 37.6 37.3
Education and Literacy		
Educational Attainment No Degree HS diploma, GED, any college		34.2 65.8
Employment and AFDC History		
Ever Worked Full-time for 6 Months or More No Yes		33.3 66.7
Earnings in Past Year No Earnings Some Earnings		79.9 20.1
Family Receipt of AFDC During Childhood No Yes		64.1 35.9
Welfare Duration Less than 2 years More than 2 years, but less than 5 years 5 years or more		18.5 36.7 44.8

Source: JOBS baseline surveys (Private Opinion Survey and Standard Client Characteristics)
Note: Calculations for this table used data for all 351 observational study respondents for whom there were baseline survey data, including experimental group members who did not participate in the JOBS Program. The sample size may fall slightly short of the number reported because of missing or unusable items from some respondents' questionnaires.

had been on welfare for less than two years, while almost half had been receiving welfare for five or more years.

Procedures and Measures

The Appendix presents a detailed summary of the measures used and, where appropriate, their psychometric properties. In this section we provide a brief description of the measures. In the welfare office, at baseline (T1), mothers provided basic demographic information and answered a brief questionnaire about attitudes. The mothers were also administered the Document Literacy sub-scale of the Test of Applied

Literacy Skills (TALS), developed by Educational Testing Service. After T1, data collection occurred through interviews in the home. Interviewers were trained to complete each interview, to administer child assessments, and to administer the mother-child teaching tasks in the observational sessions.

The measure of depressive symptoms used for the present analyses was obtained in the interview at T2 (about three months after baseline). Through a self-administered questionnaire, with interviewers providing assistance if necessary, mothers completed the Center for Epidemiological Studies Depression Scale (CES-D; Radloff, 1977).

At T3 (about five months after baseline), a videographer accompanied the interviewer for an observation of mother-child teaching tasks. The teaching tasks included a book reading and discussion task, a block task, a word guessing game task, a sorting task, and a maze task. Following these tasks the mother presented a wrapped gift to the child, with time remaining for the child to unwrap the gift.

For the analyses discussed here measures have been selected from ratings focused both on the affective quality of interactions (see Weinfield, Egeland, & Ogawa, 1998) and on the aspects of interaction related to emergent literacy (see De Temple & Snow, 1998). Both quality of relationship and mother's supportive presence, which were rated for the duration of the mother-child teaching tasks, were used as measures of an affectively positive and supportive relationship. Book reading quality (from the book reading task), ease of ideas (from the word guessing-game task), and quality of instruction (rated for the duration of the mother-child teaching tasks) were used as measures of maternal cognitive stimulation.

Two maternal report measures of parenting drawn from the interview accompanying the observational session are also examined. These measures, aggravation (which describes the mother's frustration in the parenting role) and control (which describes the mother's endorsement of physical discipline and her expectations that the child control his or her emotions rather than express them), complement the observational measures by providing the mother's perceptions of difficulty in the parenting role.

At T4 (about five years after baseline), interviewers administered a direct assessment of the child's cognitive achievement: the Woodcock-Johnson Tests of Achievement–Revised (Woodcock & Johnson, 1989, 1990). Four sub-tests were administered. The Applied Math and Calculation sub-tests were combined to create a composite Broad Math score. The Passage Comprehension and Letter-Word Comprehension sub-tests were combined to create a composite Broad Reading score. Children also answered questions about their school engagement.

Also at T4, mothers completed measures of the children's social behavior. These measures included modified versions of the Externalizing, Internalizing, and Hyperactivity sub-scales from the Social Skills Rating System (Gresham & Elliott, 1990). Mothers also answered questions regarding their children's health. These measures include a rating of the child's general health, as well as three specific questions regarding whether the child had a physical, emotional, or mental problem that required a special class or school, or that hindered the mother from working or going to school, or that required frequent medical attention.

T4 is also the source for information concerning the mother's employment status and participation in job club and/or educational activities. Mothers were asked whether they were currently working full-time for pay, whether they had worked for pay at all during the five-year follow-up period, and if they had ever participated in job club or in education or training during the five-year follow-up period. Information from unemployment insurance records also indicates the mother's current employment status at the five-year follow-up and whether she had worked for pay at all during the five-year period. In addition, we collected information at the five-year follow-up on the mother's depressive symptoms using an abbreviated version of the CES-D. A measure of recurrent depression was also created at T4. Mothers who reported high depressive symptoms at both the two- and five-year follow-ups were coded as having recurrent depressive symptoms across the follow-up period.

Strategy of Analysis

As a first step, we examine the prevalence of low literacy (measured by having scores in the two lower levels of the TALS) at baseline and moderate-to-high depressive symptoms (measured by having scores of 16 or higher on the CES-D; Devins & Orme, 1985) close to the beginning of the evaluation, in the Observational Study sample. We also examine the prevalence of the co-occurrence of moderate-to-high depressive symptoms and low literacy in the sample. Further, we note the proportion of mothers reporting current employment at the time of the five-year survey, as well as any employment over the five-year follow-up period.

In a set of two-by-two analyses of covariance we test for main effects of depressive symptoms and literacy, as well as for the interaction of these, for each dependent variable. These analyses control for the following baseline characteristics: child age, child gender, number of children in the household, marital status, race, mother's age, mother's educational level, mother's basic skills level, prior employment and earnings, prior welfare receipt, prior food stamp receipt, and research group. Since the mother's report of the child's health status and behavior problems may be subject to subjective bias from the mother, we additionally controlled for baseline depressive symptoms in these analyses. In a final set of analyses we employ structural equation modeling to examine the mediating role of parenting in explaining the effects of maternal depressive symptoms and maternal literacy on the children's math achievement and behavior problems. Specifically, we hypothesize that the relationship between child outcomes at the five-year follow-up (T4) and the measures maternal literacy (T1) and maternal depressive symptoms (T2) will be mediated by measures of parenting at T3.

FINDINGS

Prevalence of Each Potential Barrier and Their Co-Occurrence

Though these risk factors are significantly correlated, the correlation is somewhat low ($r = .19$, $p < .05$), indicating that mothers with one risk factor do not necessarily have the other. The proportion of mothers in the sample with scores indicating lower literacy (levels 1-2 on the TALS) was 52.6%. The proportion of mothers with scores indicating moderate-to-high levels of depressive symptoms (scores of 16 and higher on the CES-D) was also high: 39.5%. Nearly a quarter of the sample had a co-occurrence of lower literacy and higher depressive symptoms, while approximately a third of the mothers had neither of the potential barriers. The remainder of the mothers had only one potential barrier (28.1 percent had low literacy only, while 14.2 percent had depressive symptoms only).

Rates of Employment

At the time of the five-year follow-up, 86.0 percent of the mothers in the sample indicated that they had worked at some point during the follow-up period, and 56.2 percent indicated that they were currently employed.

Depressive Symptoms and Literacy as Predictors of Maternal Outcomes

Table 2 summarizes the results of the analyses of covariance examining the role of depressive symptoms and literacy in predicting the mother's psychological well-being, participation in job club and/or educational activities, and employment. In the analyses for maternal psychological well-being, we found that maternal depressive symptoms measured about three months after the start of the study significantly predicted depressive symptoms at the five-year follow-up, as well as recurrent depressive symptoms across the follow-up period.

Results from the analyses of maternal participation in welfare-to-work activities indicate that mothers with literacy scores in the lower two categories, indicating difficulty with functional literacy, were less likely to participate in any activities related to the program, and especially education and training activities. However, maternal depressive symptoms were not found to predict any of the participation measures. The pattern of means in Table 2 shows that mothers who were both lower in literacy and had higher depressive symptoms were the least likely to participate in any job preparation activity.

Low literacy and higher depressive symptoms were important for predicting whether these mothers were ever employed during the five years of follow-up (whether measured by maternal report or administrative records). Mothers higher in literacy were more likely to have ever been employed than mothers lower in literacy. Mothers who reported fewer depressive symptoms were also more likely to be currently employed and to report being employed at any point during the follow-up period than mothers who reported higher depressive symptoms. In addition, mothers who were both lower in literacy and higher in depressive symptoms were less likely to have ever been employed than the other mothers.

Depressive Symptoms and Literacy as Predictors of Child Outcomes

Table 3 reports the results for the analyses of covariance with respect to the child outcomes of achievement test scores, school engagement, behavior problems, and health status. Children with mothers who had higher literacy scores performed better on the achievement tests and rated themselves higher on school engagement than children whose mothers had lower literacy scores. Children whose mothers reported fewer depressive symptoms scored higher on the math achievement test

TABLE 2. Analyses of Maternal Outcomes: Main Effects and Interaction of Depressive Symptoms and Literacy

	Lower Literacy Depressive Symptoms		Higher Literacy Depressive Symptoms		F values Main Effect		
Maternal Outcome	Low Mean (SE)	High Mean (SE)	Low Mean (SE)	High Mean (SE)	Literacy	Depressive Symptoms	Interaction
Psychological Well-Being (n = 253)							
Depressive Symptoms at 5 yr follow-up	7.54(0.55)	14.72 (1.88)	6.74 (0.56)	12.48 (2.40)	1.04	16.69***	0.11
Recurrent Depressive Symptoms	0.19 (0.04)	0.62 (0.12)	0.12 (0.04)	0.52 (0.15)	0.20	20.27***	0.05
Participation (n = 283)							
Ever participated: Any activity	0.59 (0.04)[b]	0.28 (0.15)[a]	0.66 (0.04)[b]	0.80 (0.19)[b]	5.58*	0.47	3.32+
Ever participated: Job Club	0.35 (0.04)	0.12 (0.14)	0.35 (0.02)	0.44 (0.19)	1.71	0.35	1.76
Ever participated: Education/Training	0.40 (0.04)	0.20 (0.14)	0.57 (0.04)	0.74 (0.19)	7.96**	0.02	2.22
Employment (n = 283)							
Ever employed in Years 1 - 5	0.85 (0.03)[b]	0.57 (0.10)[a]	0.90 (0.03)[b]	0.90 (0.13)[b]	4.59*	2.44+	2.52+
Currently employed full time	0.53 (0.04)	0.56 (0.15)	0.59 (0.04)	0.61 (0.20)	0.17	0.05	0.00
Ever employed in Years 1- 5 (admin)	0.87 (0.03)[b]	0.63 (0.09)[a]	0.92 (0.03)[b]	0.94 (0.12)[b]	4.70*	1.93	2.60+
Currently employed (admin)	0.62 (0.04)	0.26 (0.15)	0.66 (0.04)	0.60 (0.24)	2.22	2.62+	1.42

Note. $+ p \leq .10$, $* p \leq .05$, $** p \leq .01$, $*** p \leq .001$
When an interaction is significant at $p \leq .10$, a superscript 'a' indicates where the mean of the low literacy and high depressive symptoms group is lower than the means of the other groups, while 'b' indicates means not significantly different.

TABLE 3. Analyses of Child Outcomes: Main Effects and Interaction of Depressive Symptoms and Literacy

Child Outcomes	Lower Literacy Depressive Symptoms Low Mean (SE)	Lower Literacy Depressive Symptoms High Mean (SE)	Higher Literacy Depressive Symptoms Low Mean (SE)	Higher Literacy Depressive Symptoms High Mean (SE)	F values Main Effect Literacy	F values Main Effect Depressive Symptoms	F values Interaction
Academic Functioning (n = 259)							
WJ-R - Broad Reading	91.69 (1.46) [b]	79.97 (4.74) [a]	99.39 (1.46) [b]	106.32 (6.35) [b]	17.03***	0.38	5.24*
WJ-R - Broad Math	99.82 (1.59) [b]	83.72 (5.18) [a]	105.66 (1.60) [b]	104.72 (6.94) [b]	8.86***	3.56+	2.90+
School Engagement	16.14 (0.36)	14.28 (1.17) [a]	17.22 (0.36) [b]	19.01 (1.57) [b]	8.19**	0.01	3.12+
Behavior Problems (n = 262)							
Externalizing	4.28 (0.25)	5.31 (0.83)	3.94 (0.25)	3.64 (1.11)	1.95	0.26	0.87
Internalizing	7.40 (0.29)	9.20 (0.96)	7.64 (0.29)	9.20 (1.28)	0.02	4.05*	0.02
Hyperactivity	6.01 (0.27)	7.41 (0.89)	6.09 (0.27)	7.26 (1.19)	0.00	2.75+	0.02
Health (n = 270)							
Child's General Health	4.31 (0.07)	4.08 (0.24)	4.40 (0.07)	4.55 (0.31)	1.88	0.04	0.94
Excellent/Very Good Health	0.84 (0.03)	0.74 (0.12)	0.87 (0.03)	0.83 (0.15)	0.36	0.53	0.11
Physical/Emotional/Mental Problem requiring a Special Class	0.07 (0.02)	0.20 (0.08)	0.07 (0.02)	0.02 (0.11)	1.65	0.40	1.61
Physical/Emotional/Mental Problem hindering work	0.01 (0.01)	0.09 (0.04)	0.02 (0.01)	0.01 (0.06)	1.05	1.03	1.38
Physical/Emotional/Mental Problem requiring frequent medical attention	0.06 (0.02)	-.01 (0.07)	0.05 (0.02)	0.00 (0.09)	0.01	0.94	0.03

Note. + $p \leq .10$, * $p \leq .05$, ** $p \leq .01$, *** $p \leq .001$
When an interaction is significant at $p \leq .10$, a superscript 'a' indicates where the mean of the low literacy and high depressive symptoms group is lower than the means of the other groups, while 'b' indicates means not significantly different.

77

than children of mothers reporting moderate-to-many depressive symptoms.

In addition to the findings for literacy and depression, there is some evidence that the combination of these two risk factors was important for children's academic functioning. Children whose mothers had both moderate-to-high depressive symptoms and low literacy scored lowest on the achievement tests.

The findings summarized in Table 3 show that there is some indication that maternal depressive symptoms, though not maternal literacy, were important for a child's behavior problems. Mothers with moderate-to-high depressive symptoms tended to report more internalizing and hyperactive behavior problems for their children than mothers with fewer depressive symptoms. As shown, there are no significant findings for child health status.

Parenting as a Mediator of Effects on Children's Math Achievement

To examine the role of parenting behavior in explaining the relationship between maternal depressive symptoms and low literacy with child outcomes, we selected two child outcomes: the child's math achievement and the child's behavior problems (considered as latent constructs). We limited the presentation of the structural equation models to the child's math achievement and the child's behavior problems. Structural models for the child's reading achievement scores and school engagement are similar to the models presented for the child's math achievement. Since there were no significant findings in the analyses of the child's health status, we did not pursue these outcomes in the structural models.

Figure 1 provides the structural equation model examining parenting as a mediator of maternal depressive symptoms and maternal literacy for the measure of the child's math achievement. The fit of the initially specified model of the role of parenting examining the child's math achievement was χ^2 (67, $N = 274$) = 143.98, $p < .0001$, CFI = .94, NNFI = .92, & IFI = .94, indicating that the model describes the relationships adequately. For details on the construction of the structural models, see Zaslow et al. (2001).

The model indicates, first, that both maternal literacy and maternal depressive symptoms are statistically significant predictors of multiple dimensions of parenting (see Figure 1 for standardized path coeffi-

FIGURE 1. Mediation of Child Math Achievement

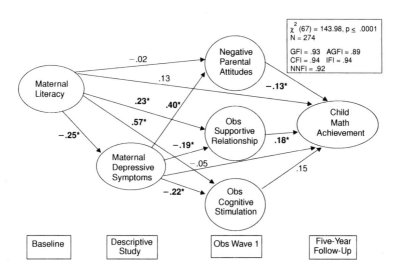

*p ≤ .05

cients). The model also indicates that the observational measure of the supportive relationship between the mother and child and the mother's negative parental attitudes mediated the effects of maternal literacy and maternal depressive symptoms on the child's math achievement. Thus, maternal depressive symptoms and maternal literacy appear to positively affect children's math achievement through the active, supportive, and reciprocal engagement that the child and mother are involved in during the observed interaction. The child's math achievement was negatively affected by maternal depressive symptoms through the mother's ratings of herself as being aggravated with parenting and more controlling of the child's behavior.

Parenting as a Mediator of Child Math Achievement for Mothers with Low and High Literacy

To answer the question of whether the pattern of mediation is different when depressive symptoms occur in the presence of lower as opposed to higher maternal literacy (see Figure 2), we estimated the model of contributors to the child's math achievement simultaneously for high

FIGURE 2. How Maternal Depressive Symptoms Function in the Presence of High and Low Literacy for Child Math Achievement

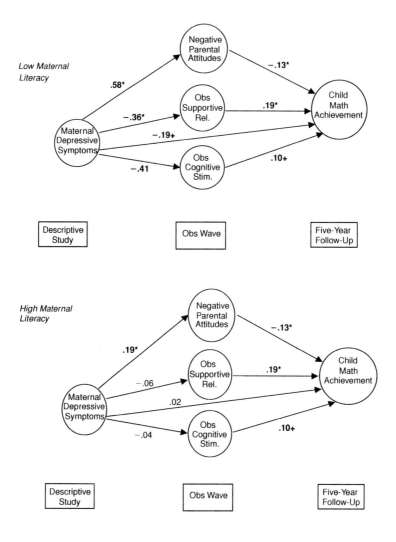

*p ≤ .05
+p ≤ .10
All numbers that show significance are in bold.

and low maternal literacy risk levels (cf., Graziano, Hair, & Finch, 1997). Estimation of the model across the literacy groups with the beta and gamma parameters free to be estimated yielded a fit of χ^2 (144, N = 274) = 269.73, p < .001. When the seven parameters in the beta and gamma matrices were set invariant across the groups, the increase in the chi-square was significant (change in χ^2 = 21.98, df change = 7), indicating that the hypothesis of invariant structural parameters could be rejected. Through a stepwise process, the parameter estimates for the effects of maternal depressive symptoms on negative parental attitudes, on the observations of supportive relationship between the mother and child, on the observational measure of cognitive stimulation, and on the child's math achievement were freed (see Figure 2). The final model was not significantly different from the model in which all the beta and gamma parameters were free to be estimated (change in χ^2 = 7.58, df change = 3).

The results indicate that the structural basis for predicting a child's math achievement is different for high and low maternal literacy. Figure 2 shows that maternal depressive symptoms are an important element in the model for low maternal literacy, with strong paths to all three parenting constructs and also mediating effects on the child's math achievement through all three parenting constructs. Even with the mediating effects of parenting, maternal depressive symptoms (in the presence of lower literacy) still have a direct negative effect on the child's math achievement. Maternal depressive symptoms do not play as important a role in the model for high maternal literacy; only one mediating effect (negative parental attitudes) on the child's math achievement was found in the presence of high maternal literacy.

Parenting as a Mediator of Effects on Children's Behavior Problems

The second model we examine is the role of maternal depressive symptoms and literacy and the mediating role of parenting for child behavior problems (Figure 3). The fit of the initially specified model of the role of parenting in mediating maternal literacy and depressive symptoms for child behavior problems is χ^2 (108, N = 267) = 194.84, p < .01, CFI = .94, NNFI = .93, and IFI = .94, indicating that the model describes the relationships adequately.

Maternal literacy and maternal depressive symptoms predicted multiple dimensions of parenting, as in the overall model for the child's

FIGURE 3. Mediation of Child Behavior Problems

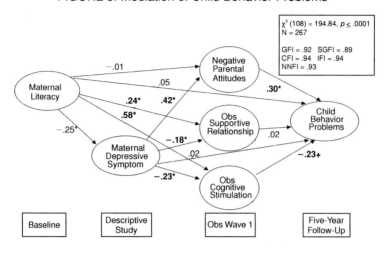

* p ≤ .05
+ p ≤ .10
All numbers that show significance are in bold.

math achievement. There is also evidence of mediation by parenting, although the particular aspects of parenting behavior that appear to be important are different for child behavior problems than for children's math achievement. Aggravated and controlling parenting was predicted by greater maternal depressive symptoms, and in turn predicted more behavior problems. At the same time, less cognitive stimulation and instruction of children by mothers was predicted by lower maternal literacy and more maternal depressive symptoms, which predicted more behavior problems in children.

Parenting as a Mediator of Child Behavioral Outcomes for Mothers with Low and High Literacy

To test whether parenting mediates the relationship of maternal depressive symptoms on children's behavior problems differently for mothers with high or low literacy (Figure 4), we estimated the model of contributors to child behavior problems simultaneously for high and low maternal literacy.

Consistent with the model for the child's math achievement, these results indicate that the structural basis for predicting child behavior prob-

FIGURE 4. How Maternal Depressive Symptoms Function in the Presence of High and Low Literacy for Child Behavior Problems

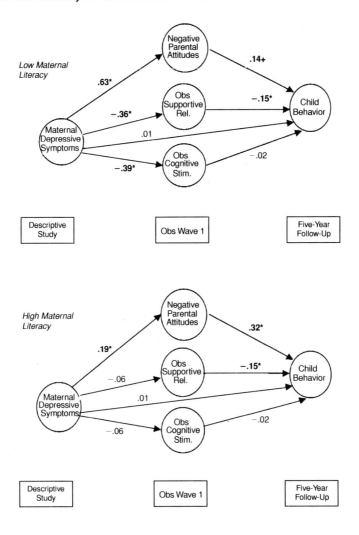

* p ≤ .05
+ p ≤ .10

lems is different for high and low maternal literacy. Estimation of the model across the literacy groups with the beta and gamma parameters free to be estimated yielded a fit of χ^2 (198, $N = 267$) = 384.80, $p < .001$. When the seven parameters in the beta and gamma matrices were set invariant across the groups, the increase in the chi-square was significant (change in χ^2 = 22.53, df change = 7), indicating that the hypothesis of invariant structural parameters could be rejected. The parameters reflecting the effects of maternal depressive symptoms on negative parental attitudes, maternal depressive symptoms on the observational measure of supportive relationship between the mother and child, maternal depressive symptoms on the observational measure of cognitive stimulation, and negative parental attitudes on child behavior problems were freed (see Figure 3). This yielded a model not significantly different from the model in which all the beta and gamma parameters were free to be estimated (change in χ^2 = 0.89, df change = 3).

Figure 4 shows that maternal depressive symptoms were a significant predictor in the model for low maternal literacy, with strong paths to all three parenting constructs. Two of the three parenting constructs (negative parental attitudes and supportive relationship) serve as significant mediators of the relationship between maternal depressive symptoms and child behavior problems in families with low maternal literacy. Maternal depressive symptoms play a different role in the model for high maternal literacy. As in the model of high maternal literacy for child math achievement, maternal depressive symptoms had a strong effect on negative parental attitudes, mediating the effect on child behavior problems.

CONCLUSION AND DISCUSSION

As welfare caseloads fall, families with greater barriers to employment may remain on the rolls. Factors that serve as barriers to employment for the parent generation can also be viewed as risks that may compromise development in the child generation. This paper examined two key barriers/risks: moderate to high maternal depressive symptoms and low maternal literacy.

The present study's findings expand the picture reported by Zaslow et al. (2001) pertaining to shorter-term employment outcomes. This previous study found lower baseline literacy to predict a lower likelihood of current employment at the two-year follow-up. There was not evidence at the two-year point that earlier depressive symptoms affected employment rates–either by themselves or in combination with low literacy. By contrast, findings from the present study indicate that mothers with both risk factors were the least likely to have ever been employed during the five-year follow-up.

Why did both low maternal literacy and greater maternal depressive symptoms appear to affect longer-term but not shorter-term employment in this sample of mothers expected to transition from welfare to work? Mothers with low literacy were less likely than their counterparts with higher literacy to have participated, even minimally (for at least a day), in some work preparation activity–and were especially less likely to have participated in basic education or training activities–at some point during the five-year follow-up period. Participation in any welfare-to-work activity was lowest for mothers with both risk factors. Thus, it would appear that the mothers who could stand to benefit the most from work preparation services–especially basic education to improve their literacy–were actually the least likely to receive these services over the five-year period. In addition, the present study found earlier depressive symptoms to predict both depressive symptoms at the five-year follow-up as well as the likelihood that mothers had relatively many depressive symptoms at both the two- *and* five-year follow-ups. It may be that the failure to obtain the services necessary for transitioning from welfare to work sustains or exacerbates already elevated levels of prior depressive symptoms, the combination of which, over time, further dampens the likelihood of finding any (let alone stable) employment.

With respect to the child generation, the present study's results both confirm and expand the findings reported by Zaslow et al. (2001), in which mothers' low baseline literacy predicted lower school readiness scores when sample children were five to seven years old. However, children's school readiness did not differ according to mothers' higher levels of depressive symptoms, either alone or in combination with low literacy. By contrast, findings from the present study, pertaining to sample children's academic achievement and engagement in school when they were between about eight and ten years old, show achievement scores and self-reported engagement to be lowest among children whose mothers had both risk factors.

The present study also found that–rather than varying by mothers' baseline literacy–children's reported behavior problems varied according to mothers' prior depressive symptoms. Unlike the findings for academic outcomes, there was no increased risk for behavior problems among children whose mothers had both risks. These findings stand in contrast to findings reported by Zaslow and colleagues for children's behavior problems when they were five to seven years old. Specifically, children whose mothers had both risks showed the worst behavior problems during these early school years yet, three years later, children whose mothers had both risks looked no different than children of mothers with only the depressive symptoms risk (though both groups of children still had more behavior problems than children whose mothers did not have elevated levels of depressive symptoms). This seems to suggest that the early years of school may somehow ameliorate the influence of low maternal literacy on behavior problems for the subgroup of children whose mothers had both risks five years earlier.

In sum, these findings, when sample children were between eight and ten years old, replicate and extend the results pertaining to these children's cognitive school readiness and behavior problems closer to school entry. Mothers' low baseline literacy predicted poorer academic outcomes at both time points, and mothers' elevated depressive symptoms close to baseline predicted poorer behavioral outcomes at both time points. Interestingly, the degree to which the co-occurrence of these maternal risks predicted the most problematic academic and behavioral outcomes for children differed for the different time periods. The co-occurrence was problematic for children's *behavior* (but not their cognitive school readiness) at school entry, and for children's *academic achievement and engagement in school* (but not their behavior problems) three years later. It may be that, for the children whose mothers have both low literacy and higher depressive symptoms, the short-term implications are behavioral, which then interferes with learning, translating into longer-term problems academically.

To what extent did parenting appear to play a role? As was found in the earlier paper, the role of parenting in mediating the effects of maternal depressive symptoms on both cognitive and behavioral outcome was apparent only, or especially, for mothers with low baseline levels of literacy. Thus, findings suggest that the effects of depressive symptoms on children's academic and behavioral outcomes are stronger in the context of low literacy or, alternatively, that higher literacy buffers children from the deleterious effects of greater maternal depressive symptoms as transmitted through parenting.

Implications for Practice and Policy

Findings from this and the previous study (Zaslow et al., 2001) suggest that low literacy and greater depressive symptoms among welfare-reliant mothers during their children's preschool years serve both as barriers to their subsequent employment, as well as serve as risk factors for their children's academic and behavioral outcomes in the elementary school years. Our findings suggest that the possibility of treating and reducing early maternal depressive symptoms may reduce the likelihood of elevated depressive symptoms years later, which may have long-term implications for these mothers' ability to seek out and successfully participate in work-preparation activities and employment. In addition, ameliorating these maternal risks would not only increase the employability of mothers but, our findings suggest, would have indirect benefits for their children. Improving mothers' literacy could improve parenting-both directly, and by buffering the negative effects of depressive symptoms on parenting-thereby improving children's academic performance both early and later on. In addition, interventions aimed at reducing mothers' depressive symptoms could diminish early behavior problems (and, consequently, later academic problems) in their children. Such improvements may be even greater for children whose mothers have low literacy.

Under prior welfare policies, mothers with many personal or family barriers to employment were exempted from mandatory participation in work preparation activities. However, with the current welfare policy's greater emphasis on work, program operators are seeking strategies aimed at increasing employability of "harder-to-employ" mothers. Human capital development strategies-gradually abandoned in the last decade in favor of "work-first" strategies-may be necessary for the lower-literacy mothers remaining in or entering today's welfare system. Research has shown that these strategies can successfully increase mothers' educational attainment (Freedman et al., 2000) and that these program-induced increases in education can bode well for children's academic and cognitive outcomes (Magnuson & McGroder, 2001; McGroder, Zaslow, Moore, & LeMenestrel, 2000). New approaches are needed, however, to encourage mothers at higher risk to engage in such programs.

Policymakers and program operators are also seeking new and creative ways to meet the needs of these "hard-to-employ" mothers-from screening for depression in welfare offices and improving the access to and funding of mental health services for low-income individuals (Lennon, Blome, & English, 2001), to screening for learning disabilities (which are likely to be quite prevalent among individuals with low literacy; Learning Disabilities Association of America, 1998), and placing learning disabled clients in supported work environments. Innovative strategies have begun to emerge (see Pavetti & Strong, 2001). Key to the success of such strategies is: (1) *program flexibility,* whereby case managers have access to a broad array of services and can tailor these services to the specific needs of multi-risk families; (2) *coordination and collaboration with other community agencies* providing mental health services and counseling for substance abuse and domestic violence, even co-location of these services in the welfare office; and (3) *the development of a trusting relationship* between case managers and these families (Pavetti, Olsen, Pindus, Pernas, & Isaacs, 1996).

While strategies to address the needs of multi-risk families in the welfare system are necessary, depression, low literacy, and characteristics that provide both other barriers to employment and risks for the family are also germane to low-income families not involved in the welfare system. Researchers and policy analysts have noted the importance of reaching out to families with multiple risks through multiple points of entry into service delivery systems, including health care (both physical and mental health), early childhood education and early intervention, and treatment for substance abuse and domestic violence (National Center for Children in Poverty, 2000).

In short, identifying mothers with multiple barriers to employment–including limited literacy and greater depressive symptoms–and targeting multiple services accordingly, may have the biggest payoff both in terms of longer-term employment outcomes for the adult generation and both shorter and longer-term outcomes for the child generation. For such multi-risk families, according to Knitzer (National Center for Children in Poverty, 2000, p. 2), "the time is right for taking a two-generational approach [because] welfare reform compels us to give attention to the adults [while] public national education goals demand we pay attention to the children." Findings in this paper, in fact, underscore the two-generational nature of risk factors in families receiving welfare and the potential importance of two-generational approaches.

REFERENCES

Administration for Children and Families. (2000). *Change in TANF caseloads since enactment of new welfare law* [On-line]. Available: http://www.acf.dhhs.gov/news/stats/aug-dec.htm.

Brooks, M.G., & Buckner, J.C. (1996). Work and welfare: job histories, barriers to employment, and predictors of work among low-income single mothers. *American Journal of Orthopsychiatry, 66*(4), 526-536.

Danziger, S., Corcoran, M., Danziger, S., Heflin, C., Kalil, A., Levine, J., Rosen, D., Seefeldt, K., Siefert, K., & Tolman, R. (1999). *Barriers to the employment of welfare recipients.* Ann Arbor, MI: University of Michigan, Poverty Research & Training Center.

Danziger, S.K., Kalil, A., & Anderson, N.J. (2000). Human capital, physical health, and mental health of welfare recipients: Co-occurrence and correlates. *Journal of Social Issues, 56* (4), 635-654.

De Temple, J., & Snow, C. (1998). Mother-child interactions related to the emergence of literacy. In M.J. Zaslow & C.A. Eldred (Eds.), *Parenting behavior in a sample of young mothers in poverty: Results of the New Chance Observational Study* (pp. 114-169). New York: Manpower Demonstration Research Corporation.

Devins, G.M., & Orme, C.M. (1985). Center for epidemiological studies depression scale. In D.J. Keyser & R.C. Sweetland (Eds.), *Test critiques* (pp. 144-160). Kansas City, MO: Test Corporation of America.

Freedman, S., Friedlander, D., Hamilton, G., Rock, J., Mitchell, M., Nudelman, J., Schweder, A., & Storto, L. (2000). *Evaluating alternative welfare-to-work approaches: Two-year impacts for eleven programs.* Washington, DC: U.S. Department of Health and Human Services, Administration for Children and Families and Office of the Assistant Secretary for Planning and Evaluation, and U.S. Department of Education.

Goodman, S.H., & Brumley, H.E. (1990). Schizophrenic and depressed mothers: Relational deficits in parenting. *Developmental Psychology, 26,* 31-39.

Graziano, W.G., Hair, E.C., & Finch, J.F. (1997). Competitiveness mediates the link between personality and group performance. *Journal of Personality and Social Psychology, 73* (6), 1394-1408.

Gresham, F.M., & Elliott, S.N. (1990). *Social Skills Rating System manual.* Circle Pines, MN: American Guidance Service.

Haveman, R., & Wolfe, B. (1995). The determinants of children's attainment: A review of methods and findings. *Journal of Economic Literature, 33,* 1829-1878.

Joreskog, K.G., & Sorbom, D. (1993). *Lisrel VIII: Structural equation modeling with the SIMPLIS command language.* Chicago: Scientific Software International.

Learning Disabilities Association of America. (1998). *Employment success for adults with learning disabilities: A resource manual for employment counselors, employers, employees, and adults seeking work.* Minneapolis, MN: Minnesota Department of Economic Security.

Lennon, M.C., Blome, J., & English, K. (2001). *Depression and low-income women: Challenges for TANF and welfare-to-work policies and programs.* New York, NY: National Center for Children in Poverty.

Magnuson, K., & McGroder, S. (2001). From ABCs to 1 2 3s: The effect of maternal education on young children's school readiness. Poster presented at the annual meeting of the Population Association of America in Washington, DC, March 29-31, 2001.

McGroder, S.M. (2000). Parenting among low-income African-American single mothers with preschool-age children: Patterns, predictors, and developmental correlates. *Child Development, 71* (3), 752-771.

McGroder, S.M., Papillo, A.R., & Zaslow, M. (2001). Maternal employment and child outcomes in welfare families. Poster presented at the annual meeting of the Population Association of America in Washington, DC, March 29-31, 2001.

McGroder, S.M., Zaslow, M.J., Moore, K.A., & LeMenestrel, S.M. (2000). *The national evaluation of welfare-to-work strategies: Impacts on young children and their families two years after enrollment: Findings from the Child Outcomes Study.* Washington, DC: U.S. Department of Health and Human Services, Administration for Children and Families and Office of the Assistant Secretary for Planning and Evaluation, and U.S. Department of Education.

McLeod, J.D., & Shanahan, M.J. (1993). Poverty, parenting, and children's mental health. *American Sociological Review, 58,* 351-366.

McLoyd, V.C. (1990). The impact of economic hardship on Black families and children: Psychological distress, parenting, and socioemotional development. *Child Development, 61*(2), 311-346.

Moffitt, R. (1999). Presentation at the Congressional Briefing, *Is welfare reform working? The impact of economic growth and policy changes.* Sponsored by the Consortium of Social Science Associations, Washington, DC.

Moore, K.A., Zaslow, M.J., Coiro, M.J., Miller, S.M., & Magenheim, E.B. (1995). *How well are they faring? AFDC Families with preschool-aged children in Atlanta at the outset of the JOBS evaluation.* Washington, DC: U.S. Department of Health and Human Services.

National Center for Children in Poverty (2000). Helping vulnerable young children affected by welfare reform. *News & Issues, Vol. 10, No. 2,* pp. 1-2. New York, NY: National Center for Children in Poverty.

Olson, K., & Pavetti, L. (1996). *Personal and family challenges to the successful transition from welfare to work.* Washington, DC: The Urban Institute.

Panter, A.T., Tanaka, J.S., & Hoyle, R.H. (1994). Structural models for multimode designs in personality and temperament research. In C.F. Halverson, G.A. Kohnstamm, & R.P. Martin (Eds.), *The developing structure of temperament and personality from infancy to adulthood* (pp. 111-138). Hillsdale, NJ: Erlbaum.

Pavetti, L., Olsen, K., Pindus, N., Pernas, M., & Isaacs, J. (1996). *Designing welfare-to-work programs for families facing challenges: Lessons from the field.* Washington, DC: The Urban Institute.

Pavetti, L., & Strong, D. (2001). *Work-based strategies for hard-to-employ TANF recipients: A preliminary assessment of program models and dimensions.* Washington, DC: Mathematica Policy Research.

Radloff, L.S. (1977). The CES-D scale: A self-report depression scale for research in the general population. *Applied Psychological Measurement, 1,* 385-401.

Seefeldt, K. (2001). Presentation in the session on Identifying Barriers to Work at the Fourth Annual Welfare Reform Evaluation Conference, sponsored by the Administration for Children and Families. Arlington, VA, May 22-24, 2001.

Weinfield, N.S., Egeland, B., & Ogawa, J.R. (1998). The affective quality of mother-child interactions. In M.J. Zaslow & C.A. Eldred (Eds.), *Parenting behavior in a sample of young mothers in poverty: Results of the New Chance Observational Study.* New York: Manpower Demonstration Research Corporation.

Woodcock, R.W., & Johnson, M.B. (1989, 1990). *Woodcock-Johnson Psycho-Educational Battery–revised.* Allen, TX: DLM Teaching Resources.

Zaslow, M.J., Hair, E., Dion, M.R., Ahluwalia, S., & Sargent, J. (2001). *Maternal depressive symptoms and low literacy as potential barriers to employment in a sample of families receiving welfare: Are there two-generational implications?* Manuscript submitted for publication.

Zaslow, M.J., McGroder, S.M., Cave, G., & Mariner, C. (1999). Maternal employment and child outcomes among families with some history of welfare receipt. In R. Hodson (Series Ed.) & T. Parcel (Vol. Ed.), *Research in the Sociology of Work: Vol. 7, Work and Family* (pp. 233-259). Stamford, CT: JAI Press.

APPENDIX. Description of Measures Used in the Present Analyses

Category/Variable	Wave of Data	Description
Independent Variables		
Maternal Literacy	T1	Assessed using the Test of Applied Literacy Skills (TALS), document literacy scale. Developed by Educational Testing Service. Yields measure of broad reading skill in everyday life, such as ability to use information in tables, schedule, charts, maps and forms. Scores are divided into 5 levels. Scores in levels 3, 4, or 5 indicate ability to integrate pieces of information or to disregard irrelevant information in documents. Levels 1 and 2 indicate difficulty in performing tasks that require integration of information from various parts of a document.
Maternal Depressive Symptoms	T2	Assessed using Center for Epidemiological Studies Depression Scale (CES-D). The CES-D is a widely used measure of depressive symptomatology designed for use in the general population (Radloff, 1977). Respondents indicate the frequency in the past week of feelings such as sadness, loneliness, difficulty sleeping, lack of appetite). Scores of 16 or higher out of a possible 60 indicate a moderate to high level of depressive symptoms, and have been found to distinguish between clinically depressed patients and others (Devins & Orme, 1985). Internal consistency reliability in the present sample was high (Cronbach's alpha of .86). In the present analyses, scores above 16 were used to indicate moderate to high depressive symptoms.
Dependent Variables: Mother's Report of Psychological Well-Being		
Depressive Symptoms at the Five-Year Follow-Up	T4	Twelve items from the 20-item CES-D Scale (Radloff, 1977) were used to measure depressive symptomatology at the five-year follow-up. Respondents rated how often in the past week: *"I was bothered by things that usually don't bother me." "I did not feel like eating; my appetite was poor." "I felt that I could not shake off the blues even with help from my family or friends." "I had trouble keeping my mind on what I was doing." "I felt that everything I did was an effort." "I felt fearful." "My sleep was restless." "I talked less than usual." "I felt lonely." "I felt sad." "I could not get going." "I felt depressed."* Respondents rated the frequency as: Rarely (less than 1 day), Some (1-2 days), Occasionally (3-4 days), Most (5-7 days).

APPENDIX (continued)

Category/Variable	Wave of Data	Descripton
Recurrent Depressive Symptoms Over the Follow-Up Period	T4	Respondents were categorized as having recurrent depressive symptoms if they were categorized as having moderate to high symptoms at both the two-year and the five-year follow-ups.
Dependent Variables: Mother's Report of Maternal Employment		
Any Maternal Employment During the Five-Year Follow-Up	T4	Mothers reported whether they had been employed at all since random assignment.
Current Maternal Employment	T4	Mothers reported whether they were currently working for pay.
Any Maternal Employment During the Five-Year Follow-Up (Administrative Records)	T4	Mothers were categorized as having any employment since random assignment if they were employed during any quarter in years 1 through 5.
Current Maternal Employment (Administrative Records)	T4	Mothers were categorized as being currently employed if they were employed in the last quarter of year 5.
Dependent Variables: Mother's Report of Participation in Work Preparation Activities		
Participated in Any Activity	T4	Mothers' responses to items about participation in job club, education, or training since random assignment were collapsed to obtain the measure of participation in any activity.
Participated in Job Club	T4	Mothers were asked, "Since (RAD), have you ever attended classes or gotten assistance that lasted for a few weeks on preparing resumes and job applications, or calling employers?" This activity is sometimes called "job club" or "job search."
Participated in Education/Training	T4	Mothers' responses to items about education or training since random assignment (for example, ESL classes, college courses, or vocational training classes) were collapsed to obtain the measure of participation in any education/training.
Dependent Variables: Child Outcomes: Academic Functioning		
Woodcock-Johnson Tests of Achievement–Revised: Broad Reading Score	T4	Focal children were administered the Passage Comprehension and Letter-Word Identification tests. Composite score is age-standardized, with a mean of 100 and a standard deviation of 15.
Woodcock-Johnson Tests of Achievement–Revised: Broad Math Score	T4	Focal children were administered the Calculation and Applied Problems tests. Composite score is age-standardized, with a mean of 100 and a standard deviation of 15.
School Engagement	T4	Focal children rated themselves from 0 to 3 on seven items measuring school engagement, where 0 = "never true," 1 = "sometimes true," 2 = "often true," and 3 = "very often true." Summary scores range from 0 to 21. The items are: "When I'm in school, I feel happy." "I work very hard in school." "When I'm in school, I feel bored." "When I'm in school, I pay attention in class." "I try to learn as much as I can about my school subjects." "When I'm in class, I just pretend to work." "When I'm in class, I try very hard."

APPENDIX (continued)

Category/Variable	Wave of Data	Description
Dependent Variables: Child Outcomes: Mother's Report of Behavior Problems		
Externalizing Behaviors	T4	Includes such behaviors as fighting and arguing with others. Possible scores range from 0 to 18.
Internalizing Behaviors	T4	Behaviors such as acting sad and being anxious about being with others. Possible scores range from 0 to 24.
Hyperactivity	T4	Includes such behaviors as disrupting others and acting without thinking. Scores could range from 0 to 18.
Dependent Variables: Child Outcomes: Mother's Report of Health		
General Health Rating	T4	"Would you say that your child's health in general is: (1) Excellent, (2) Very good, (3) Good, (4) Fair, (5) Poor?"
In Very Good/Excellent Health	T4	Responses to the general health rating item were dichotomized so as to obtain the measure of whether the focal child was in very good or excellent health.
Physical/Emotional/ Mental Problem Requiring a Special Class or School	T4	"(Does your child/Do any of your children) go to a special class or special school, or get special help in school for any physical, emotional, or mental condition?"
Physical/Emotional/ Mental Problem Impeding Mother's Ability to Go to School or Work	T4	"(Does your child/Do any of your children) have a physical, emotional, or mental condition that demands a lot of your attention and makes it hard for you to go to school or work?"
Physical/Emotional/ Mental Problem Requiring Frequent Medical Attention	T4	"(Does your child/Do any of your children) have a physical, emotional, or mental condition that requires frequent medical attention, frequent use of medication, or the use of any special equipment such as a wheelchair or a breathing mask?" It was specified that this does not include eyeglasses.
Mediating Variables: Maternal Report Parenting Measures		
Control	T3	Mother indicated level of agreement on a scale of 0 to 10 (10 indicating strong agreement) on five items indicating attitudes toward use of physical punishment and emphasis placed on emotional self-control (e.g., "I teach my child to keep control of his or her feelings at all times," and "It is sometimes necessary to discipline with a good, hard spanking."). Cronbach's alpha in the present sample of .63. Measures were standardized with a mean of zero.
Aggravation	T3	Mother indicated level of agreement on a scale of 0 to 10 (10 indicating strong agreement) on nine items describing feelings of stress and frustration in the parenting role. Items were taken and sometimes adapted from the Parenting Stress Index (Abidin, 1986). Examples of items on this scale: "I find myself giving up more of my life to meet my child's needs than I ever expected" and "I would be doing better in my life without children." Cronbach's alpha in the present sample of .65. Measures were standardized with a mean of zero.

APPENDIX (continued)

Category/Variable	Wave of Data	Description
Mediating Variables: Observational Measures of Parenting		
Supportive Presence	T3	Rating across full set of mother-child teaching tasks, reflecting the degree to which the mother is emotionally supportive and encouraging toward her child during the structured tasks. This rating had a potential range from 1 to 7, with higher scores indicating more supportiveness (Weinfield, Egeland & Ogawa, 1998). Interrater reliability for this rating was high, with an intraclass correlation of .79.
Quality of Relationship	T3	Rating across full set of mother-child teaching tasks, reflecting the affective and behavioral reciprocity of the mother-child relationship. This rating had a potential range of 1 to 7, with a higher score indicating greater relatedness and mutual engagement, with conflicts readily and amicably resolved (Weinfield, Egeland & Ogawa, 1998). Interrater reliability for this rating was high, with an intraclass correlation of .78.
Quality of Instruction	T3	Rating across the full set of mother-child teaching tasks, with a potential score of 1 to 7. This rating "evaluates how well the mother structures the situation so that the child knows what the task objectives are and receives hints or corrections" while solving the problems" that are timely and well-paced, provided in a progression that the child can follow, and stated clearly (Weinfield, Egeland & Ogawa, 1998, p. 78). Interrater reliability for this rating was high, with an intraclass correlation of .77.
Book Reading Quality	T3	Rating based on observation of maternal behavior during the book reading task. A composite of three ratings (each with a possible range of 1 to 3): Intonation and Animation, Comfort Level, and Fluency. Composite could range from 3 to 9, with a higher score indicating better quality book reading. The ratings were completed by one coder, and reviewed by an experienced coder. Discrepancies were discussed with a third coder until consensus was reached (De Temple & Snow, 1998).
Ease of Ideas	T3	Rating based on observation of maternal behavior during the word guessing game task. Range of 1 to 4, with a higher score denoting a better understanding and use of effective strategies to get the child to name as many wheeled objects as possible. Ratings were completed by one coder, and reviewed by an experienced coder. Discrepancies were discussed with a third coder until consensus was reached (De Temple & Snow, 1998).

Notes. T1 is at baseline, the time of enrollment in the study, with data collected prior to random assignment.
T2 is at the time of the Descriptive Study, completed approximately two to three months after baseline.
T3 is at Wave 1 of the Observational Study, completed on average five months after baseline.
T4 is data from the five-year follow-up of the Child Outcome Study of the NEWWS evaluation.

Providing Financial Empowerment to Mothers on Welfare: Pilot Evaluations of a Hospitality Training Program

Joseph R. Ferrari
Adriana Gracia
Adriana Morales

DePaul University

SUMMARY. Three samples of urban Latina and African-American women in hospitality training programs were assessed on their perceived self-efficacy. In Sample 1, the typical Latina ($n = 25$) and African-American ($n = 71$) woman was a young, single, mother of three children who had received benefits for over six years and who, at the start of a two-week training program, reported low self-efficacy and moderate so-

Address correspondence to: Joseph R. Ferrari, Department of Psychology, DePaul University, 2219 North Kenmore Avenue, Chicago, IL 60614 (E-mail: jferrari@ depaul.edu).

The authors express much gratitude to the students, instructors, and staff at DePaul's Office of Applied Innovations for their cooperation in the process of this study, especially Mary Gallagher and Tippi Reed for continued support and assistance.

These projects were part of Senior Honor's Theses by the second and third authors with the guidance of the first author. Portions were presented at the 1999 annual meeting of the *Eastern Psychological Association* (Samples 1 and 3), Providence, RI, and the 1999 biennial meeting of the *Society for Community Research and Action* (Sample 2), New Haven, CT.

95

cial desirability. Sample 2 participants were mostly single Latina ($n =$ 25) or African-American ($n = 49$) mothers who received six weeks of training/internship, but reported no significant change in their level of self-efficacy, social desirability, or hopefulness from pre- to post-training. Sample 3 (16 Latinas, 36 African-Americans) was a subset of women from the first sample who were interviewed by telephone four months after completing the two-week training program and were now employed. These working women reported a significant increase in their level of self-efficacy compared to the start of training. Results suggest that some minority women may benefit from job skill training in terms of their sense of mastery over their life situation, although the impact of such training may not emerge until after they have been actively employed. *[Article copies available for a fee from The Haworth Document Delivery Service: 1-800-HAWORTH. E-mail address: <getinfo@haworthpressinc. com> Website: <http://www.HaworthPress.com> © 2002 by The Haworth Press, Inc. All rights reserved.]*

KEYWORDS. Self-sufficiency, job training, welfare reform

It is estimated that 39 million people in the United States are "economically poor," and 3.5 million of these persons are families receiving federal assistance in the form of welfare payments (Seecombe, James, & Walters, 1998). From 1973 to 1993, the number of families living below the poverty level headed by single mothers increased from 11.5% to 25.9%, while the number of children raised solely by single mothers increased by over 50% (Lichter, McLaughlin, & Ribar, 1997). In 1996, the United States Congress replaced nearly 60 years of welfare entitlement with the current, more punitive program that made women and women with children personally responsible for their economic survival (Brooks & Bucker, 1996; Riemer, 1997a). Under a new federal law, welfare recipients are required to work in order to receive benefits and may receive those benefits up to a five-year lifetime limit (Piotrkowski & Kessler-Skiar, 1996). Although support for child care is offered under this new law, services are no longer guaranteed. These changes are reflected in the name now given to federal assistance: "Temporary Aid to Needy Families" (TANF), rather than "Aid to Families with Dependent Children" (AFDC).

The major goal of TANF is to reduce welfare dependence in each state to set goals, with 25% of welfare recipients per state to have been employed by 1997 (Seecombe et al., 1998), increasing to 50% employed by 2002 (Franklin, 1998). In short, the objective of TANF is to promote a sense of "financial empowerment" among recipients by placing them in jobs of 30 hour per week or more, while assisting families in caring for children in a home-like environment (Franklin, 1998).

Many states adopted a "work-promotion model" which emphasized education and training to facilitate a quick entry of welfare recipients into the labor force, even if often in low-level jobs (Riemer, 1997b). Under TANF, states were granted the right to create programs tailored to their individual needs and preferences as long as they followed certain provisions of federal law. Federal funding to the state was provided through block grants that offered fixed amounts without regard to the unemployment rates or per capita incomes of state residents. Working, then, within the constraints of money on the one hand and federal provisions on the other, each state could determine the style and focus of its job training.

According to the U. S. Department of Health and Human Services, 90% of adult welfare recipients are women; 37% of welfare recipients are African-Americans, while 25% are members of other minority populations, including Hispanics (U. S. Dept. of Health & Human Services, 1993). However, in the state of Illinois women of color comprise a larger percentage of the caseload of welfare recipients than ever before (Grumman, 1999). Today, 79% of welfare recipients are non-Caucasian (compared to 75% in 1998 and 73% in 1997). Furthermore, demographic information suggests that the "typical" welfare person of color was a woman, age 25 or older, with at least one to two children (Coll, Surrey, & Weingarten, 1998). The woman had been the financial head of the household since being divorced, was now single, and often the family had received government assistance for three years (Coll et al., 1988). In terms of life history on welfare, it appears that most welfare mothers were themselves persons raised by single heads of household mothers on welfare (Duncan, Hill, & Hoffman, 1988).

TANF has not had the same impact on minority families as it has had on families of white ancestry. Since June, 1997, the number of white families on welfare dropped from 50,796 to 25,631–a drop of nearly 50%. Meanwhile, the number of minority families fell from 140,331 to 97,938, a decrease of nearly 30%. Furthermore, persons living in downstate Illinois have moved off the state's welfare program at almost double the rate of recipients in Cook county, where the city of Chicago is located. As of July, 1999, within the greater Chicago area approximately 36.6% of Hispanic and 27.7% of African-American families receiving welfare, compared to 41.7% of the white families, have found employment and moved off the recipient list.

The present study focused exclusively on women of color who were recipients of welfare in the city of Chicago, Illinois. We assessed persons living in Chicago in order to gain a profile of women from a large metropolitan setting who were moving off welfare. We focused on women of color (Latina and African-American) in order to assess the impact of job training programs on those women most likely to be affected by welfare reform. These minority samples represent groups of economically disadvantaged persons who were the least likely served by the federal reforms in the welfare program (Brooks & Buckner, 1996; Grumman, 1999; Riemer, 1997a; Salomon et al., 1996; Taylor, Casten, & Flickinger, 1993).

To assess the impact of training programs on mothers who had been receiving AFDC, and now TANF, support, we focused on the psychological construct of *self-efficacy*. Self-efficacy is the belief that one can bring about a desired outcome through one's own actions (Bandura, 1977; 1997). The focus here is on the belief that a certain task can be performed, rather than the measured level of performance that determines whether a certain task has been fulfilled. Changes in one's level of self-efficacy may occur through having formerly succeeding in accomplishing a task, observing others who have succeeded at a task, being convinced that one can accomplish a task, and reducing fears and apprehensions associated with not being able to accomplish a task (Bandura, 1997). Perceived self-efficacy pertains to optimistic beliefs about being able to cope with a variety of stressors and about one's competence to deal with challenging encounters (Bandura, 1997; Maddux, 1995: Schwarzer, 1992). Sterrett (1998) demonstrated that small group job training with a sample of 900 unemployed persons could produce effective positive changes in levels of self-efficacy. Instruction focused on ways to seek jobs and to present oneself to prospective employers at the interview phase. Self-efficacy ratings increased from before to after the job-skills training program. Wolfe, Nordstrom, and Williams (1998), however, found that training which promoted self-efficacy on a particular skill among 90 newly hired telemarketers did not produce improved job performance. Actual skills recorded at the end of training were not judged to be superior to those of a control group of participants who did not receive self-efficacy training. These two studies seem inconsistent about the effects of job training to increase a person's perceived self-efficacy. It is possible that participants in the Wolfe et al. (1998) study were not provided enough opportunity to fully change or develop their sense of self-efficacy. Participants in Sterrett (1998) may have received greater levels of social and tangible support (e.g., rides to/from their job, day care) that assisted in their sense of optimism or hopefulness, as well as self-efficacy.

We explored whether a job training program improved the general perceived self-efficacy among welfare African-American and Latina women with children and a personal history of living on welfare. These women began and completed job skill training; some received an internship experience as part of training. We also included a measure of hopefulness with one sample of participants in order to obtain a more well-rounded sense of future optimism. It is possible that participants who come to believe that their economic life will change through job training and subsequent employment may become more hopeful about their future quality of life. Thus, it is possible that the perceived self-efficacy of women moving off welfare increases, as Bandura (1977; 1997) claimed, only after having direct experience with the task, receiving social support before, during, and after training, and observing peers successfully become "financially empowered" (Jarrett, 1996; Riemer, 1997b; Sansone, 1998).

DEPAUL'S OFFICE OF APPLIED INNOVATIONS AND THE HOST PROGRAM

In 1996 the "Office of Applied Innovations" (OAI), an independent Chicago-area non-profit agency affiliated with DePaul University, was created. One of its major goals was to obtain local, state and federal financial support to create and develop welfare-to-work training programs for the urban poor, then assist graduates from that program to find placement in entry-level jobs that promote financial empowerment.

One of the programs developed by OAI that had both the largest enrollment and highest rate of job placement was the "Hospitality Occupational Skills Training" (HOST) Program. In this program clients developed job-readiness skills such as effective interviewing and services associated with the hotel industry. The services they learned included such skills as how to greet hotel guests, respond to their needs, clean and service hotel guest rooms, and perform as a clerk or cashier at a hotel. Training also included life and employment skills such as stress regulation, study skills, financial budgeting, establishing credit, completing job applications, writing resumés, personal hygiene, dressing for interviews and employment, following supervisor directions, and job punctuality.

Originally, HOST training consisted of two weeks of daily meetings with clients focusing on the development of job-readiness skills such as resumé writing, interview behaviors, and application completion. Students received instruction on corporate terminology associated with the hotel industry, as well as the skills and tasks needed to work effectively in hotels. OAI realized, however, that a brief two-week HOST training program did not accomplish all their goals to promote "financial empowerment" (i.e., economic self-sufficiency). Classroom training expanded to four weeks. Additional training included discussions concerning the enhancement of self-esteem and various practices aimed at enriching customer satisfaction, practice at effective responses to customer conflicts and complaints, and reflection on ways to work constructively with employers. A two-week internship, with pay, was also added. Clients were given the opportunity to spend time at a hotel working as an intern in order to gain actual experience and while continuing to practice and enhance their newly acquired skills. The internship exposed participants to a job site, which aided in the transition to the workplace while it still permitted OAI staff and peers to provide social and emotional support. During their internship women received $25.00 a week for daily expenses (e.g., transportation and lunch).

This study presents the results of an assessment of the psychological sense of self-efficacy by Latina and African-American women clients who entered and completed the HOST program. We expected that the longer the training program (i.e., two-weeks vs. six-weeks) the greater the likelihood that self-reported self-efficacy would increase, regardless of the racial or ethnic identity of the participants. However, we also thought that persons with a long history of living on welfare may not show much improvement in their sense of self-efficacy after just a few weeks of training. It was possible that the greatest likelihood of increasing a person's self-efficacy may come from the combination of training followed by actual time spent employed on a job. A third sample of participants were interviewed by telephone four months after they finished training. During the interview these new employees were asked questions about their present employment situation, as well as re-administered the self-efficacy scale.

SAMPLE 1:
MOTHERS IN A TWO-WEEK TRAINING PROGRAM
TO LEAVE WELFARE

Research indicates that the "typical" welfare recipient has been a woman, age 25 or older, who may have a high school education, divorced and single, with at least one or two children (Coll et al., 1998). Sample 1 was assessed to learn more about "who" the typical client was who was being served by the HOST training initiative. There were no a priori expectations about the results of the training program, but we did believe that the participants would report relatively low levels of self-efficacy.

METHOD

Participants

All participants in the HOST program were Latina and African-American women who were required by TANF regulations to seek job-skill training and move off welfare. Participants volunteered for this study, were assured of the complete anonymity and confidentiality of their responses, and did not receive payments for participating. Every participant signed and dated a consent form prior to completing the demographic information.

Procedure. Participants were asked to volunteer for this study after being assured that it was independent of the training program and their eligibility for TANF support. The data were collected by the second and third authors, who are bilingual in English and Spanish. To accommodate clients with English as their second language, all items were translated into Spanish, then retranslated back to English to check for accuracy. All data were collected at the first or second HOST training class meeting with clients, at the start of class, in groups of 15 to 20 per class. Approximately 30-40 minutes were required to permit participants to complete the forms and measures, then hold a brief discussion of the purpose of the study.

If they agreed, participants returned a signed and dated consent form and completed a set of demographic items, six rating scales about their needs or expectations concerning the program and subsequent employment, and two standard psychometric measures. Demographic items provided us with a complete profile of urban women with children who participated in the HOST program. These items included their age, race or ethnicity, marital status, number of children, level of education and history of experience with the welfare program (in terms of both family background and their own years of participation). Six rating scales (1 = *strongly disagree*; 5 = *strongly agree*) were administered at the start of the training program (pre-training) and again at the end of the training program at the last meeting class (post-training). These items included: (1) I believe the training program is (was) good and worthwhile; (2) Knowing that there are similar others on welfare is (was) reassuring; (3) I have a need for day care when working; (4) The location of a job site is very important to me; (5) Learning to use public transportation is (was) very important to my employment; and, (6) I believe I will find a job after this program.

The first psychometric test participants completed before receiving HOST training was the General Perceived Self-Efficacy Inventory, a 10-item survey that uses 5-point scales (1 = *not at all true*; 5 = *very true*) (Schwarzer, 1992). We chose this inventory because it is parsimonious, has had extensive use with international samples, and has been translated into over 13 different languages, including Spanish. Sample items include "When I am confronted with a problem, I can usually find several solutions" and "Thanks to my resourcefulness, I know how to handle unforeseen situations." The self-efficacy inventory has been used in numerous studies and typically yields internal consistencies between .75 and .91, with a mean score between 20.3 and 33.5. In the present sample coefficient alpha was .84 and the mean score was 29.8 (SD = 5.2). Convergent and discriminative validity studies have indicated that scores on the self-efficacy inventory correlate positively with self-esteem and negatively with anxiety, depression, and physical symptoms (Schwarzer, 1994).

Before beginning their HOST training, participants also completed the 33-item, True/False Marlowe-Crowne Social Desirability Inventory (Crowne & Marlowe, 1960). The social desirability measure was included to assess whether participants tended to provide socially appropriate answers to our questions, such as perceived self-efficacy. Sample items include "I'm always willing to admit my mistakes" and "I have almost never felt the urge to tell someone off." Crowne and Marlowe (1960) reported that the scale has good internal consistency with varied samples (.73 to .88) and temporal stability (.84 to .88), with a mean score of 15.5 (SD = 4.4). In Sample 1, the coefficient alpha was .79 with a mean score of 18.21 (SD = 5.9).

RESULTS AND DISCUSSION

Demographics

Table 1 presents the demographic profile of Latina and African-American women in Sample 1. Chi-square and *t* tests showed no significant

TABLE 1. Number and Highest Percentage, or Mean Value, on Demographic Variables for Latina and African-American Women in Sample 1

Demographic Variable	Latina (n = 25)				African-American (n = 71)			
	n	High %	M	SD	n	High %	M	SD
Age (in years)			31.89	7.89			32.99	6.99
Marital Status								
Single	19	76%			53	75%		
Married	3				9			
Divorced or separated	3				9			
Number of Children			2.76	1.88			2.89	1.41
Education								
Elementary school	3				8			
Some high school	7				20			
High school/G.E.D.	12	48%			35	49%		
Some college	2				3			
College	0				1			
Trade school/diploma	1				4			
History of Public Assistance								
Length of time (years)			8.04	4.62			8.22	6.88
Family history								
Mother	17	68%			48	68%		
Father	0				1			
Sister(s)	6				18			
Grandparent(s)	2				4			

differences between these two sets of women on each of the demographic variables. As indicated in Table 1 the typical person entering the hospitality training program offered by DePaul's OAI was a woman in her early 30s (M = 32.1 years old), single (75.5%), with approximately three children (M = 2.9 children), who had a high school degree or less (88.4%). Furthermore, these young single mothers had spent a number of years on welfare (M = 8.2 years) and had themselves grown up with a mother (68%), and frequently a sister (24.7%), also on welfare. In short, these urban women with children mirror the typical profile of the "welfare mom" reported in previous program evaluations (Brooks & Buckner, 1996; Moore & Driscoll, 1997; Salomon et al., 1996).

Program and Employment Items

A mixed ANOVA with repeated measures was conducted to compare the training and employment needs of Latina and African-American participants. There was no significant difference between these two groups of women with children at the beginning or end of the two-week training on any of these scales. Overall, participants in the two-week training program believed the program was somewhat worthwhile (pre, $M = 2.8$, $SD = 1.5$; post, $M = 2.8$, $SD = 1.7$), felt relatively reassured knowing that there were similar others (pre, $M = 3.7$, $SD = 1.2$; post, $M = 4.0$, $SD = 1.3$), held a consistent need for day care while working (pre, $M = 3.7$, $SD = 1.2$; post, $M = 3.7$, $SD = 1.4$), sensed a continued desire for a job in a preferred location (pre, $M = 3.7$, $SD = 1.3$; post, $M = 3.9$, $SD = 1.3$), wanted to know how to use mass transit to/from work (pre, $M = 4.1$, $SD = 1.0$; post, $M = 4.0$, $SD = 1.3$), and had a relatively consistent belief that they would find a job after the training program (pre, $M = 4.0$, $SD = 1.1$; post, $M = 3.9$, $SD = 1.6$). Thus, it appears that these participants did not report the two-week program having a major impact on their financial empowerment.

Psychometric Inventories

We examined the relationship between self-efficacy and social desirability among the participants (see Table 2 for mean scores). *T* tests comparing Latina and African-American participants on the self-efficacy and social desirability scales indicated that, at the start of training, there were no significant differences in their mean scores on social desirability and self-efficacy. However, when racial and ethnic categories were collapsed, there was a significant negative correlation between self-efficacy and *SD*, $r = -.35$, $p < .04$. The more self-efficacy participants reported the less of a tendency there was to report socially desirable responses.

We also correlated pre-training social desirability and self-efficacy scores with pre- and post-training ratings on the six program scales. At the start of the training program, self-efficacy ratings were significantly positively related to a sense of reassurance in knowing that there were similar others on welfare, $r = .33$, $p < .01$. At the completion of the program, self-efficacy ratings were significantly related to a belief that the training was good and worthwhile, $r = .43$, $p < .001$, and that they would find a desirable job, $r = .69$, $p < .001$. None of these scales were significantly related to pre-training social desirability scores.

TABLE 2. Scores on Social Desirability and Self-Efficacy for Latina and African-American Women, and Matched Comparison Groups, in Sample 1

	Social Desirability			Self-Efficacy		
	M	SD	[alpha]	M	SD	[alpha]
Present Sample						
Latina (n = 25)	18.3	3.5		28.5	4.5	
			[.79]			[.84]
African-Americans (n = 71)	18.3	4.9		29.3	4.3	
Crowne/Marlowe's Sample (1960)						
Students (n = 300)	15.5		[.78]	NA		
Schwarzer's Sample (1992)						
Costa Rican (n = 602)	NA			33.0	4.9	[.81]

Note. NA = Not Available

We then compared the pre-training mean scores on the social desirability measure between our sample of women with children who were receiving welfare support and a sample of college women, with a mean age of 21, reported by Crowne and Marlowe (1960). T tests for these independent groups found significant differences in *SD* between Crowne and Marlowe's (1960) sample and the present samples of Latina women, t (323) $= -6.99$, $p < .001$, and African-American women, t (625) $= -9.44$, $p < .001$. Both the Latina and African-American women in the present study reported higher levels of social desirability than non-welfare recipient, young adults. These results suggest that women on welfare in Sample 1 may have had a stronger desire to provide us with socially appropriate responses to our questions. Of course, this comparison is between two groups that are very different in terms of time of testing, age and many other background factors. Nevertheless, it may serve to indicate the level of mistrust participants in welfare training programs have when they participate in activities that are presented to them as "research studies."

Finally, we compared pre-training self-efficacy scores within the two sets of welfare participants (Latina and African-American) with a "matched" sample of women (see Table 2) reported by Schwarzer (1992). Schwarzer (1992) reported international data collected in a number of countries across varied races and ethnic identifications but there was only one group that was an appropriate "matched" comparison of adult Spanish women (*M* age = 22 years old). These women lived in Costa Rica. T tests for independent groups found a significant difference in self-reported self-efficacy between Schwarzer's (1992) Spanish sample and the present samples of Latina welfare women, $t(625) = 10.37$, $p < .001$, with the welfare women reporting lower levels of self-efficacy than the non-welfare women. Unfortunately, there was no comparison group of African-American women with or without children who completed the self-efficacy scale.

Taken together these results suggest, at most, that the welfare women with children in Sample 1: (a) did not differ significantly among themselves in their reported tendency toward social desirability and perceived self-efficacy; (b) as a total group, may have been more prone toward socially desirable responding; and, (c) if they are Latina, may report lower self-efficacy than other Hispanic women. These data offered an initial profile of participants in the DePaul HOST training program.

SAMPLE 2: EXPLORING CHANGES IN SELF-EFFICACY AND HOPEFULNESS BEFORE AND AFTER TRAINING

It appears that the participants in the two-week HOST program were "typical" of welfare women with children, but they did not expect financial empowerment from such a brief program of training. We evaluated the revised six-week HOST programs, again comparing Latina and African-American women. As with the first sample, we inquired about demographic background and asked about perceived sense of self-efficacy and social desirability. For Sample 2 we also assessed their overall hopefulness about their futures. Hopefulness was assessed because we wanted to examine the beliefs participants had about their present and future opportunities in life. We believed that including both self-efficacy and hopefulness with this sample would make it possible to examine in closer detail the impact welfare-to-work programs have on the optimism of women with children.

METHOD

Participants

All participants in the HOST program were either Latina ($n = 25$) or African-American ($n = 49$) women who were required, in order to receive temporary TANF funding, to gain job-skill training and seek to leave the welfare system. However, all participants were assured that involvement in the study's data collection process would not affect their funding support. None of these women were in the two-week training program, and all participants volunteered for the present study by signing and dating a consent form.

Procedure

As with Sample 1, data were collected by the second and third authors, and to accommodate clients for whom English was their second language, all items were translated into Spanish, then retranslated back to English to check for accuracy. All pre-training data were collected at the first or second meeting with clients at the start of the HOST training classes and all post-internship data were collected on the last day of class. Testing occurred in groups of 15 to 20 per class, with participants requiring about 45 minutes to complete all items.

All participants completed the set of demographic items (age, race, marital status, number of children, education level, and personal/family history on welfare). Five rating-scale items using 5-point scales focused on program evaluation and employment needs, as in Sample 1: (1) a belief that the training program is (was) worthwhile, (2) awareness of others in a similar situation is reassuring/comforting, (3) the location of the job site is personally important, (4) a need for day care when working is personally important, and (5) a belief that one will be (is) able to find a job. We added two pre- and post-training scales about the program and employment needs: "The internship experience is (was) worthwhile," and "The overall training program is (was) satisfying," along with two items administered only prior to training: "Receiving health benefits is important for my employment," and "Receiving paid vacation benefits is important for my employment." Finally, we also asked participants to tell us the number of hours it took them to arrive at both the training class and to their internship/new job experience, the number of miles they traveled to work, the number of day care sites they knew of in their local community, the number of days per week they spent looking for a job, which days of the week (Monday through Sunday) they spent looking for a job, and which days of the week they most often obtained an interview for employment.

All participants completed, at both pre- and post-training survey sessions, Schwarzer's (1992) self-efficacy inventory, the 33-item Marlowe-Crowne social desirability scale, and Snyder, Harris, Anderson, Holleran, Irving et al.'s (1991) 12-item, 8-point Hope Scale. Snyder et al. (1991) claimed that hopefulness is a cognitive set based on a reciprocally derived sense of successful determination on two scales, one based on meeting one's goals (termed "agency"; sample item, "I've been pretty successful in life") and one based on being able to generate successful paths to meet those goals (termed "pathways"; sample item, "I can think of many ways to get out of a jam"). An overall sense of hopefulness is obtained by summing the scores of both the agency and pathway scales. The mean score and coefficient alpha with the present sample on the self-efficacy inventory was 30.9 (SD = 4.7) and 0.79, the social desirability scale was 17.7 (SD = 4.3) and 0.85, and the overall hopefulness scale was 23.7 (SD = 3.9) and 0.75, respectively.

RESULTS AND DISCUSSION

Demographics

Chi-square and t tests were performed on the demographic profile items for the 16 Latina and 36 African-American women in Sample 2. There were no significant differences between these two sets of women on the demographic variables. The typical person entering the six-week hospitality training program was a woman in her early 30s (M = 31.9 years old), single (72.7%), with three children (M = 3.0 children), and a high school degree or less (86.4%). These young mothers had spent, on average, 7.3 years on welfare (SD = 5.1) and often had a mother who had been on welfare (48%). Thus, these women were similar to the participants in Sample 1 and participants described in other research on welfare programs (e.g., Jennings & Krane, 1998; Salomon, Bassuk, & Brooks, 1996).

Ratings on Pre- and Post-Program and Employment Items

Table 3 presents the mean ratings on the set of pre-and post-training program and employment items. The analysis employed a mixed ANOVA with repeated measures to assess differences among the nine training program and employment needs with respect to Latina and African-American participants. Overall, there were no significant differences on most of the items between these two sets of women at the start or end of the six-week training and internship program. However, there

TABLE 3. Ratings of Training Program Items by Latina and African-American Women in Sample 2

Program Item		Latina (*n* = 25)		African-American (*n* = 49)	
		Pre-training	Post-training	Pre-training	Post-training
Interview Training	M	4.1	4.8	4.5	4.2
is/was Worthwhile	SD	1.3	0.6	0.8	1.2
Awareness of Similar	M	3.8	4.7	4.0	4.1
Others is/was Comforting	SD	1.2	0.8	1.3	1.3
Day Care Availability	M	3.2	4.4	4.0	4.2
is Important for a Job	SD	1.5	1.3	1.4	1.1
Job Location is Important	M	4.2	4.8	4.1	3.9
for Deciding to Work	SD	1.0	0.9	1.0	1.2
Self-Confident will be/am	M	4.8	4.6	4.6	4.4
Able to Find a Job	SD	0.6	0.7	0.8	0.9
Internship Experience	M	4.6	4.8	4.4	4.7
is/was Worthwhile	SD	0.9	0.7	0.9	0.8
Overall Job Program	M	4.7	4.8	4.5	4.4
is/was Worthwhile	SD	0.8	0.6	0.9	0.9
Health Benefits	M	4.8	NA	4.5	NA
are Important for a Job	SD	0.6		0.9	
Paid Vacation Benefits	M	4.6	NA	4.2	NA
are Important for a Job	SD	0.8		1.0	

Note. Scale range: 1 = "not at all," 5 = "very much." NA = Not Available.

was a significant difference between Latina and African-American women in pre- to post-training ratings of the perceived importance of day care availability for a job, $F(1, 50) = 6.6, p < .05$, and the location of the job, $F(1, 50) = 7.8, p < .01$. At the start of the training program Latina welfare moms gave the least importance to the availability of day care, but at post-training showed the greatest increase in the perceived importance of day care. Also, compared to African-American women, Latina women at post-training indicated that the location of the job site was very important in deciding whether to accept a job offer. Together, these results indicate that there are personal employment issues which may differentiate the concerns of minority women on welfare.

In addition, we conducted *t* tests for independent groups between Latina and African-American women on the other employment need items. There were no significant differences between the two sets. Participants reported traveling, on average, 1.6 hours to reach the training site, 33.4 minutes to travel to their new job site, and about 20 miles to reach that site. Participants reported knowing that there were, on average, 1.8 local day care sites in their neighborhood. Also, participants spent an average of 2.1 days per week looking for a job (usually Mondays, Wednesdays, and Tuesdays, in that order), and were actually interviewed on Tuesdays and Thursdays. These results indicate that travel times, distance to and from work, and day care availability were all important issues to minority women moving off welfare, and that these women did spend time actively seeking full-time employment.

Pre- and Post-Training Scores on Psychometric Inventories

To assess changes in self-efficacy, hopefulness, and social desirability scores from pre- to post-training, we performed mixed ANOVAs with repeated measures on each of these scores for Latina and African-American participants across the two measurement sessions. There were no significant differences between the two sets of women with respect to either their pre- or post-training scores. Collapsing across the two sets of women, for Self-Efficacy participants reported a mean of 33.19 ($SD = 5.01$) at pre-training and 33.80 ($SD = 4.73$) at post-training. For the Hope scale, participants reported a mean of 23.71 ($SD = 3.95$) at pre-training and 26.00 ($SD = 3.73$) at post-training. For the social desirability measure participants reported a mean of 27.34 ($SD = 5.67$) at pre-training and 29.54 ($SD = 4.77$) at post-training.

It appeared, then, that the six-week training program (which included an on-the-job internship) did not produce significant increases in personal self-efficacy or in overall hopefulness in the future. These results were surprising (and discouraging) since they suggest that the present welfare job training program did not produce measurable changes in the sense of mastery and optimism for the future among two sets of minority women. However, they are consistent with Wolfe et al. (1998) who found that job training may not produce changes in perceived self-efficacy. Together with the two-week training program reported with Sample 1, it seems that OAI's hospitality program did not produce significant personal perception changes with Latina and African-American mothers moving off welfare.

We also correlated self-efficacy, hopefulness, and social desirability scores at pre- and post-training. Social desirability and self-efficacy ratings were not significantly related at the start of training, $r = .02, p > .10$, nor at the end of training, $r = .05, p > .10$. Similarly, social desirability and hopefulness were not significantly related at the start, $r = .13, p >$

.10, nor at the end of training, $r = .12$, $p > .10$. However, self-efficacy and hopefulness were significantly related at both the start, $r = .79$, $p < .01$, and end, $r = .73$, $p < .01$, of training. These results are encouraging, because they demonstrate that the responses to standardized psychometric inventories were not confounded by social desirability tendencies at either pre- or post-training. Moreover, they suggest that self-efficacy and hopefulness (our measure of optimism) were related constructs. Participants who claimed high self-efficacy at the start of the training program also reported similar tendencies at the end of training.

SAMPLE 3:
FOLLOW-UP INTERVIEW WITH WORKING WOMEN

One may not be all that surprised with the lack of increase in reported self-efficacy found in Samples 1 and 2 above. Both sets of women, for both samples, reported long life histories of being on welfare. Most participants reported growing up with a welfare mother, and they themselves had been living on welfare with their children for a number of years. It is possible that brief intervention training programs do not produce immediate changes in personal self-efficacy (cf. Wolfe et al., 1998). Receiving just a short set of job skills is not enough to change perceptions of low financial empowerment (Riemer, 1997a; 1997b). Therefore, we conducted a brief, four-month follow-up phone interview with participants from Sample 1. A four-month follow-up was selected because it would provide respondents enough time to adjust to continued employment and to reflect on their personal sense of accomplishment since the end of the HOST training program. We chose participants in Sample 1 instead of those in Sample 2 because of convenience and the larger sample size. Also, if reported increases in self-efficacy occur with women who only received a two-week training program, then it is quite possible that greater increases may occur with working women who received an even longer training program.

During the phone interview, interviewers asked employment questions and re-administered the self-efficacy scale. We decided not to re-administer all the measures over the phone for practical reasons: we did not want psychological reactance or negative affect by respondents to arise because of a long and lengthy phone interview; also, we did not have the financial resources to conduct lengthy phone interviews.

METHOD

Participants

The demographic profile for the women included in Sample 3 (16 Latina, 36 African-American) did not differ significantly from the population of women from which they were drawn, and they did not differ significantly from each other. Across the participants in Sample 3, most women were young (M age = 31.2), single (74%), the mother of about three children (M = 2.77), and had a high school degree or less (87.1%). These women had been on welfare an average of 7.7 years (SD = 4.8) and often had grown up with a mother on welfare (49%).

Procedure

The second author contacted participants using telephone numbers provided by OAI. She made a series of four phone calls (in the day and evening; during the week and weekends) to reach participants in order to conduct the interview. She was unable to contact 44 persons from Sample 1 (45.8% of the total sample) due to no answer (47.4%), disconnected phones with no forwarding numbers (35.3%), wrong numbers listed with the OAI (6.8%), no known phone number (6.0%), or because the person had moved without a forwarding number (3.8%). Once a participant was contacted, the interviewer reminded the woman about her involvement with DePaul's HOST training program and the previous data collection process. She then asked if the participant would volunteer for a brief follow-up interview over the telephone, asking questions about her current employment and her self-efficacy perception.

All the women reached by phone agreed to participate in the phone interview. Each participant was then asked to report: (a) the number of jobs held since completing training; (b) number of months at the present job; (c) hourly and weekly wage from their current job; (d) number of hours worked per day and per week; and, (e) their overall satisfaction (on a 5-point rating scale: 1 = *very unsatisfied,* 5 = *very satisfied*) with their fringe benefit package from their current employer. We chose these few items because they provided a general profile of the current employment profile of these former welfare recipients. Also, participants were asked to complete Schwarzer's (1992) 10-item self-efficacy scale.

RESULTS AND DISCUSSION

From among those women who participated in Sample 1, we were able to reach by phone 64% of the Latina and 50.7% of the African-American women. *T* tests for independent groups were performed on the set of employment items for both samples of women. There were no significant differences on these items. Across participants, these working women reported that they had held 1.2 jobs in the past four months (*SD* = 0.84), had been at the present position for 2.0 months (*SD* = 0.82), currently earned $6.94 per hour (*SD* = $1.45) and $284.75 per week (*SD* = $34.33), worked 7.5 hours per day (*SD* = 1.73) and 29.80 hours per week (*SD* = 13.14). Participants also stated that they were not particularly satisfied with their overall employment fringe benefit package (*M* = 2.50, *SD* = 0.71). Taken together, it seems that these former welfare mothers were not making especially high wages (the wages reported were slightly higher than the minimum wage) or in a state of strong financial empowerment four months after completing job training. Possibly, the four-month follow-up period was not enough time to demonstrate a significant change, and the fact that participants were only employed with their current employer for two months did not enable participants to earn high wages.

In addition, we examined the reported social desirability scores between these Latina and African-American women, then compared those participants reached by phone (*n* = 52) with those persons not reached by phone (*n* = 44). Table 4 presents the mean score on social desirability at pre- and post-training for Latina and African-American women in Sample 3. *T* tests for independent groups indicated that there were no significant differences between these two sets of women at either their pre- or post-training scores, and *t* tests for correlated groups suggested no significant change in scores from pre- to post-training for either set of women. In addition, *t* tests for independent groups indicated no significant difference in social desirability scores between participants reached by phone (*M* = 21.5) and those persons not reached by phone (*M* = 19.1). These results suggest that the Latina and African-Americans interviewed by phone four months following completion of training were not significantly different in their tendencies toward socially desirable responses among themselves nor when compared to people we were unable to interview. Such results provide us with confidence that our analyses were not compromised by the confounding variable of social desirability in responses.

TABLE 4. Pre-Training, Post-Training, and Follow-up Measures for Latina and African-American Women in Sample 3

Sample and Measure		Measurement Session		
		Pre-training	Post-training	Follow-up
Latinas (n = 16)				
Self-efficacy	*M*	28.6	31.8	32.6
	SD	4.8	5.4	4.9
Social desirability	*M*	21.3	21.2	NA
	SD	5.7	5.9	
African-Americans (n = 36)				
Self-efficacy	*M*	34.4	33.1	35.0
	SD	3.8	5.0	3.6
Social desirability	*M*	22.3	25.0	NA
	SD	4.5	4.5	

Note. NA = Not Available.

Further, we used pre-training, post-training, and follow-up measurements to conduct mixed ANOVAs with repeated measures on self-efficacy scores for Latina and African-American participants in Sample 3. Table 4 presents the mean scores on self-efficacy across measurement sessions for Latinas and African-Americans. There was a significant difference in self-efficacy between these sets of women at pre-training, $F(1, 50) = 10.30, p < .004$, and again at the follow-up phone interview, $F(1, 50) = 4.33, p < .05$, with African-Americans claiming higher self-efficacy than Latina women at both measurement sessions. Moreover, there was a significant increase from pre-training to follow-up for Latina women in self-efficacy, $F(1, 50) = 6.73, p < .03$. Newman-Keuls post hoc comparisons indicated that the difference lay in pre-training scores compared to follow-up scores. Based on these results, it appears that the African-American women in Sample 3 did not show a significant change in their perception of self-efficacy across measurement sessions. Perhaps their higher scores throughout the sessions reflected a "ceiling effect" in that they started and remained so high in their perceived self-efficacy that they had little chance for variability. In contrast, the Latina participants did report a significant increase from their initial scores to their follow-up scores. For these individuals, working and earning even a small amount of income reflected a change in their perceptions of self-efficacy.

In summary, the results from Sample 3 participants suggest that working mothers who had participated in a brief job training program did not seem to be making a large amount of money several months after "graduation." Their demographic profile was similar to other participants in this study and other reported research on low-income, working mothers (e.g., Brooks & Buckner, 1996; Franklin, 1998; Riemer, 1997a). However, for Latina, if not African-American working mothers, after working for several months there was an increase in their sense of self-efficacy, an effect independent of social desirability. This finding may seem surprising, given the low daily and weekly wages earned at their full-time job. Nevertheless, the positive impact of employment after training (i.e., financial empowerment) seems to provide a sense of personal gain or merit to at least some categories of minority women.

GENERAL CONCLUSION

This study reported information about urban minority mothers who received job training to help them leave welfare. The demographic profiles of the women in our samples matched those of persons cited in other published research (e.g., Duncan et al., 1988; Lichter et al., 1997; Salomon et al., 1996). Participants in the present study received a job training program for entry level positions in the hospitality field. Interviews with women who completed the program and had been working for several months in the field indicated that their weekly pay was low and the fringe benefits less than optimal, findings also similar to those reported in other studies of working poor women (Jarrett, 1996). As Riemer (1997b) states, the current forms of job training for welfare persons are "quick fixes" that may not substantially improve their quality of life. We found support for this claim in the lack of changes in overall hopefulness in life reported by women in Sample 2. The skills that welfare recipients may obtain did not seem to move them into "financial empowerment." Future job training program development is needed for at least urban women of color.

In contrast, the results from Sample 3 do suggest some promising avenues for future research. Several months after they began work there seemed to be gains in perceived self-efficacy among Latina women, though not African-American women. It is important to note that these levels of self-efficacy were not associated with personal desire for social approval. It may be that African-American women started their association with the HOST program at a higher level of self-efficacy than the Latina women and there was little room for variability. It is also possible that the personal perceptions of African-American women are different than those of other women of color (Jarrett, 1996; Taylor et al., 1993), and future research may want to explore those individual ethnic differences. Nevertheless, it is interesting to note that changes in perceived self-efficacy occurred for Latina women only after they had been actually working at their new job. Wolfe et al. (1998) failed to find significant changes in self-efficacy after a training program, yet Sterrett (1998) did report such changes. The present study suggests that change in perceived self-efficacy may occur in a "sleep effect" for some individuals. That is, change does not immediately occur after training but only gradually, after spending time in actual employment. Future research with working urban minority mothers who have histories as welfare recipients is needed. We suggest that job-training programs for welfare recipients focus on the long-term implications of their initiatives. The true impact of their effects may not be immediate, but appear only after time.

REFERENCES

Bandura, A. (1977). Self-efficacy: Toward a unifying theory of behavioral change. *Psychological Review, 84*, 191-215.

Bandura, A. (1997). *Self-efficacy: The exercise of control.* New York: Freeman.

Brooks, M., & Buckner, J. (1996). Work and welfare: Job histories, barriers to employment, and predictors of work among low-income single mothers. *American Journal of Orthopsychiatry, 66*, 526-537.

Coll, C.G., Surrey, L.A., & Weingarten, A. (1998). *Mothering against the odds: Diverse voices of contemporary mothers.* New York, NY: Guilford Press.

Crowne, D.P., & Marlowe, D. (1960). A new scale of social desirability independent of psychopathology. *Journal of Consulting Psychology, 24*, 349-354.

Duncan, G.J., Hill, M.S., & Hoffman, S.D. (1988). Dependence within and across generations. *Science, 239*, 467-471.

Franklin, S. (1998). Welfare rolls to payrolls. *The Chicago Tribune Newspaper,* pp. 20-23.

Grumman, C. (1999: June 27). Welfare caseloads slashed in 2 years: But system still not serving needs of all recipients. *The Chicago Tribune Newspaper,* pp. 1, 11.

Jarrett, R.L. (1996). Welfare stigma among low-income African-American single mothers. *Family Relations, 45*, 368-374.

Jennings, W.T., & Krane, D. (1998). Inter-organizational cooperation and the implementation of welfare reform: Community service employment in welfare work programs. *Policy Studies Review, 15*, 170-201.

Lichter, D.T., McLaughlin, D.K., & Ribar, D.C. (1997). Welfare and the rise in female-headed families. *American Journal of Sociology, 103*, 112-143.

Maddux, J. (1995). *Self-efficacy, adoption, and adjustment: Theory, research, and application.* New York: Plenum.

Moore, K., & Driscoll, A. (1997). Low-wage maternal employment and outcomes for children: A study. *The Future of Children, 7,* 122-127.

Piotrkowski, C., & Kessler-Skiar, S. (1996). Welfare reform and access to family-supportive benefits in the workplace. *American Journal of Orthopsychiatry, 66,* 538-547.

Riemer, F.J. (1997a). From welfare to working poor: Prioritizing practice in research on employment-training programs for the poor. *Anthropology and Education Quarterly, 28,* 85-110.

Riemer, F.J. (1997b). Quick attachments to the workforce: An ethnographic analysis of a transition from welfare to low-wage jobs. *Social Work Research, 21,* 225-232.

Salomon, A., Bassuk, S., & Brooks, M. (1996). Patterns of welfare use among poor and homeless women. *American Journal of Orthopsychiatry, 66,* 510-525.

Sansone, F.A. (1998). Social support's contribution to reducing welfare dependency: Program outcomes of long term welfare recipients. *Journal of Sociology and Social Welfare, 25,* 105-126.

Schwarzer, R. (1992). *Self-efficacy: Thought control of action.* Washington, DC: Hemisphere.

Schwarzer, R. (1994). Optimism, vulnerability, and self-beliefs as health-related cognitions: A systematic overview. *Psychology and Health: An International Journal, 9,* 161-180.

Seecombe, K., James, D., & Walters, K.B. (1998). "They think you aren't much of nothing": The social construction of the welfare mother. *Journal of Marriage and the Family, 60,* 846-865.

Snyder, C.R., Harris, C., Anderson, J.R., Holleran, S.A., Irving, L.M., Sigmon, S.T., Yoshinobu, L., Gibb, J., Langelle, C., & Harney, P. (1991). The will and the ways: Development and validation of an individual-differences measure of hope. *Journal of Personality and Social Psychology, 60,* 570-585.

Sterrett, E.A. (1998). Use of a job club to increase self-efficacy: A case study of return to work. *Journal of Employment Counseling, 35,* 69-78.

Taylor, R., Casten, R., & Flickinger, S. (1993). Influence of kinship social support on the parenting experiences and psychosocial adjustment of African-American adolescents. *Developmental Psychology, 29,* 382-388.

U.S. Department of Health and Human Services (1993). *Characteristics and financial circumstances of AFDC recipients.* Washington, DC: U.S. Government Printing Office.

Wolfe, S.L., Nordstrom, C.R., & Williams, K.B. (1998). The effects of enhancing self-efficacy prior to job training. *Journal of Social Behavior and Personality, 13,* 633-650.

Career Search Efficacy
Among an At-Risk Sample:
Examining Changes
Among Welfare Recipients

Irene J. Franze
Joseph R. Ferrari
DePaul University

SUMMARY. Since the introduction of welfare reform more job training programs have become available to welfare recipients; however, these programs rarely undergo thorough assessments of their effectiveness in improving the psychological well-being of participants. The purpose of this study was to examine how career search efficacy may change among welfare ($n = 14$) and non-welfare recipients ($n = 27$) enrolled in a 10-week work training program that included classroom instruction, job simulation practice, and an internship. Results suggested that both welfare and non-welfare recipients improved on two career search efficacy factors (interviewing and network efficacy) from the start to end of the training program. *[Article copies available for a fee from The Haworth Document Delivery Service: 1-800-HAWORTH.*

Address correspondence to: Joseph R. Ferrari, Department of Psychology, DePaul University, 2219 North Kenmore Avenue, Chicago, IL 60614-3504 (E-mail: jferrari@.depaul.edu).

The authors express much gratitude to Mary Gallagher, Rosie Carter, Stephanie Frangola, and Tippie Reed at OAI for support in conducting this study.

Partial funding for this project was made available by DePaul University's Office of Applied Innovations (OAI).

[Haworth co-indexing entry note]: "Career Search Efficacy Among an At-Risk Sample: Examining Changes Among Welfare Recipients." Franze, Irene J., and Joseph R. Ferrari. Co-published simultaneously in *Journal of Prevention & Intervention in the Community* (The Haworth Press, Inc.) Vol. 23, No. 1/2, 2002, pp. 119-128; and: *The Transition from Welfare to Work: Processes, Challenges, and Outcomes* (ed: Sharon Telleen, and Judith V. Sayad) The Haworth Press, Inc., 2002, pp. 119-128. Single or multiple copies of this article are available for a fee from The Haworth Document Delivery Service [1-800-HAWORTH, 9:00 a.m. - 5:00 p.m. (EST). E-mail address: getinfo@haworthpressinc.com].

E-mail address: <getinfo@haworthpressinc.com> Website: <http://www. HaworthPress.com> © 2002 by The Haworth Press, Inc. All rights reserved.]

KEYWORDS. Welfare reform, job readiness, self-sufficiency

According to Chartrand and Rose (1996) the privilege of strategizing and selecting a career is often reserved for those from advantaged socioeconomic backgrounds, while rarely available to those from at-risk backgrounds. Perhaps a challenge in meeting the career development needs of at-risk populations lies in the fact that very little information exists regarding the psychological well-being of those in need. Chartrand and Rose (1996) suggest that this is particularly true for racial and ethnic minorities.

The current labor market, on the other hand, demands advanced technical skills and knowledge. At-risk populations, such as welfare recipients, are often unable to obtain gainful employment in the present marketplace because they are unskilled. In fact, research suggests that even in time of economic growth in the United States, the unemployment rates among African-Americans are 2.5 times greater than that of Caucasians (Swinton, 1992). This is not surprising considering that African-Americans have been found to possess lower career expectations (Hughes & Demo, 1998).

Additionally, at-risk populations lack adequate education and work experience, which is especially evident among long-term welfare recipients. In fact, research suggests that among female welfare recipients 63% have less than a high school degree and 50% have no practical work experience (Pavetti, 1995). Strategies that may increase the employability of welfare recipients must include techniques that facilitate searching for and obtaining employment, provide education and training, and create financial incentives.

In the years since the introduction of welfare reform more training programs have become available for welfare recipients than ever before. However, these programs rarely undergo thorough assessments to examine their effectiveness with respect to the process of change in the program's participants. Thus, little is known about the cognitive and emotional well-being of welfare-to-work recipients as a result of training. In fact, even less is known about the participants' beliefs regarding their capabilities to successfully perform important tasks related to the career search and selection process–a concept known as *career search efficacy* (Solberg, Good, & Nord, 1994).

According to Bandura (1977), the concept of self-efficacy refers to an individual's positive belief that he or she is capable of effectively organizing and implementing a strategy essential to performing a task. Bandura's construct of self-efficacy has been used to understand career development and career-related behaviors (Hackett & Betz, 1981). This is not surprising, since self-efficacy offers a framework for comprehending factors associated with an individual's degree of effectiveness in performing tasks essential for procuring a job (Solberg et al., 1994). Bandura (1977, 1986) claims that efficacy development is contingent not only on individual factors, but environmental factors as well. For example, Solberg et al. (1994) recommends that career assistance providers should be responsible for creating opportunities that foster the career search efficacy development.

Bandura (1986) suggests that four types of self-efficacy experiences foster a learning environment and aid in the development of self-efficacy expectations. These efficacy experiences are: (1) *enactive attainment,* which is an individual's mastery experience that is directly related to a specific task; (2) *vicarious experiences,* which result from observing others who are similar and perform a given task effectively; (3) *verbal persuasion,* which involves words of encouragement and general verbal feedback to the person attempting a specific task; and (4) *emotional arousal,* which is the physiological result of stress, anxiety, and/or depression.

Solberg et al. (1994) recommends that Bandura's (1986) self-efficacy experiences be utilized by career development professionals when creating programs to promote and develop career self-efficacy. These researchers suggest that interventions and training programs that utilize a combination of efficacy experiences can be expected to be even more effective than programs that do not make use of these experiences.

To assess the degree of career search efficacy among those seeking careers/jobs, changing careers/jobs, or reentering the job market, Solberg, Good, and Nord (1991) developed the "Career Search Efficacy Scale" (CSES). The CSES assesses four aspects (or factors) of career search efficacy: (1) *job search efficacy,* which refers to job search tasks such as identifying potential employers, managing societal and personal barriers, and understanding one's skill set; (2) *interviewing efficacy,* which involves a variety of interviewing tasks such as evaluating job requirements and preparing for interviews; (3) *network efficacy,* which consists of networking tasks such as utilizing social networks and soliciting assistance from established professionals; and (4) *personal exploration efficacy,* which involves examining career values and preferences.

While it is still not known who can benefit most from career search efficacy training, Solberg et al. (1994) claims that at-risk populations would benefit from interventions intended to increase self-efficacy. Some of these at-risk populations include members of ethnic minorities, individuals from disadvantaged backgrounds, and women seeking non-traditional employment. To date, there has not been an intervention program which focuses explicitly on developing or improving the career search efficacy of welfare recipients. In fact, only one study examined the career search efficacy of a similar at-risk sample, and results suggested an improvement in the self-efficacy of welfare recipients as a result of their participation in a "job club" (Sterrett, 1998). Hence, the present study examines how the career search efficacy of an at-risk sample (participants in a welfare-to-work training program) changed during a 10-week training program. It was hypothesized that both at-risk welfare and non-welfare recipients would improve their career search efficacy as a result of participating in training that incorporated career search efficacy experiences.

METHOD

Participants

Participants were adult (*M* age = 33.10; *SD* = 11.06) women (*n* = 26) and men (*n* = 19) enrolled in one of three 10-week long training courses offered from September, 1999 to July, 2000. Most participants self-identified as either African-American (58.1%), Hispanic (34.9%), Caucasian (2.3%), or other (4.7%) as their ethnicity. The majority of the participants (48.8%) were single, with an average of 1.91 children. Also, some participants (31.1%) reported themselves to be recipients of Temporary Assistance to Needy Families (TANF), while the remaining participants were unemployed individuals from disadvantaged backgrounds.

Research Site

This study was a field investigation of a training and development program offered through DePaul University's "Office of Applied Innovations" (OAI). The program was called "Community Kitchens" with a primary mission to provide low-income, disadvantaged individuals with employable job skills in the food service industry. OAI is funded solely by external grants, contracts and fee-for-service programs through federal, state and private sources. The OAI Community Kitchens program was staffed by 11 full-time instructors, supervisors, and clerical employees.

The Community Kitchens program trained clientele in the following areas: (1) cooking skills, (2) nutrition basics, (3) sanitation, (4) health and safety, (5) time and stress management, (6) job readiness, (7) personal finance, and (8) goal setting. Participants trained for a total of 10 weeks, four of which included classroom instruction and kitchen skills plus six weeks at an off-site internship.

Psychometric Measures

Participants completed Sterrett's (1998) *Modified Career Search Efficacy Scale (MCSES),* a valid and reliable measure of career search efficacy of adults who are interested in finding careers/jobs, changing careers/jobs, or reentering the job market. This 35-item, 7-point scale (1 = not at all confident, 7 = very confident) was used to assess the degree of confidence an individual possesses for performing career search efficacy tasks (Solberg, Good, Nord, & Holm et al., 1994). This measurement assesses four principle factors: (a) job exploration, (b) interviewing, (c) networking, and (d) personal exploration efficacy. Items include "How confident are you in your ability to develop realistic strategies for locating and securing employment? " and "How confident are you in your ability to utilize your social networks to gain employment?" Reliability estimates utilizing Cronbach's alpha were 0.97 for the full scale and ranged between 0.85 and 0.95 for each of the sub-scales (Solberg et al., 1993, as cited in Solberg et al., 1994). In the present study, coefficient alpha wave was 0.97 (full scale: M score = 7.36), 0.96 (job search efficacy: M score = 7.41), 0 .90 (interviewing efficacy: M score = 7.24), 0.90 (networking efficacy: M score = 7.22), and 0.91 (personal exploration: M score = 7.7). It should be noted that the *MCSES* is a version of the *Career Search Efficacy Scale* (Solberg et al., 1991). The *MCSES* was modified by Sterrett (1998) to serve those with an approximate seventh-grade reading level. We used this revised *MCSES* to ensure the readability levels of the participants.

Procedure

Participants were asked by the first author to volunteer for this study and were assured that their confidential participation would not affect their training or eligibility for public assistance. The researcher provided a five-minute explanation of the data collection process before the participants signed and dated a consent form. Subsequently, participants completed demographic items (e.g., age, gender, marital status, number of children), then completed the MCSES. Participants took approximately 30 to 40 minutes to complete the measure.

Each participant completed the MCSES twice during the 10-week training program. The initial data-collection wave occurred on the first day of the class prior to class instruction, and the second data-collection wave took place on the last day of class.

A typical week in the Community Kitchen program involved equipping participants with skills and knowledge necessary to procure a job in the food industry. For example, one week was committed to the interviewing process. The interview training was broken down into three themes: (1) verbal expression, (2) proper behavior and attire, and (3) stress management. This training utilized all four self-efficacy experiences to enhance the participants' learning. For example, the participants engaged in role play scenarios and mock interviews. During these activities, participants were encouraged to give each other feedback on their performance. The participants also partook in relaxation exercises to aid in detecting and managing their stress reactions during an interview. Additionally, the participants spent part of the day in a kitchen developing skills and knowledge related to cooking, nutrition and sanitation.

RESULTS

Dependent sample t-tests were performed to determine if the participants' career search efficacy from the beginning to the end of the training program changed significantly. Analysis of the full scale scores suggest that training did in fact improve the participants' career search efficacy, $t(16) = 2.39, p < .05$. As noted in Table 1, at the start of training, participants reported a total MCSES score of 250.82 ($SD = 46.57$), and at the end of training reported an increased mean score of 281.58 ($SD = 54.02$).

Results also showed that participants improved on two factor subscores: interviewing efficacy, $t(42) = 23.229, p < .05$, and networking efficacy, $t(18) = 3.524, p < .05$. Table 1 indicates that interviewing efficacy and networking efficacy increased from the start to the end of the training program. However, similar increases only approached sig-

TABLE 1. Mean Sub-Score on Factors of the Career Search Efficacy Scale at the Beginning and End of the Training Program

Career Search Efficacy Scores:		Testing Session	
		Start (n = 41)	End (n = 17)
Networking efficacy	M	55.63	63.42
	SD	11.19	9.66
Interviewing efficacy	M	50.95	57.95
	SD	11.40	12.97
Job search efficacy	M	50.55	55.23
	SD	10.07	11.73
Personal exploration efficacy	M	40.23	45.82
	SD	23.49	13.17
TOTAL SCALE SCORE	M	250.82	281.58
	SD	46.57	54.02

nificance for job search efficacy, $t(16) = 1.949, p = .06$, and were not significant for personal exploration efficacy, $t(16) = 1.047, p = .33$.

To determine if there was a difference in self-efficacy scores between welfare and non-welfare recipients from the start to the end of training, a one-way, repeated measures ANOVA was performed. Results showed a significant difference on the networking factor, $F(1, 16) = 5.04, p < .05$; non-welfare recipients showed greater improvement ($M = 64.55; SD = 11.18$) than welfare recipients ($M = 55.33; SD = 14.35$). No significant differences were found on the other three career search efficacy factor sub-scores.

To determine if career search efficacy changed from the start to the end of the training for men and women in the welfare conditions, a 2 (gender: male versus female) × 2 (group: welfare versus non-welfare recipients) mixed ANOVA, with repeated measures on the first and last measurement waves, was conducted. Results indicated no significant main or interaction effects for gender and welfare status on any of the four career search efficacy factors nor the full MCSES.

DISCUSSION

The present findings suggest that welfare-to-work training programs that incorporate Bandura's (1986) self-efficacy experiences may aid in the development of self-efficacy expectations for this at-risk sample. Career self-efficacy improvement occurred for two out of the four career self-efficacy factors with this sample, specifically interviewing efficacy and networking efficacy. This improvement is more than likely a result of the extensive training in interviews and networking offered by this program. The factors that did not yield a significant change were personal exploration efficacy and job search efficacy, although the latter did approach significance ($p < .06$). It is possible that individuals from disadvantaged backgrounds find themselves seeking blue-collar employment which often may not encourage employees to explore their personal values as these pertain to career preferences and career development. Therefore, personal exploration efficacy would not improve. Alternately, for this at-risk population OAI trainers in the present program may have neglected to include training specifically directed at personal exploration. Training instead emphasized other basic job skills that participants lacked, particularly those that involve interviewing, resumé writing, and networking. As for career search efficacy, lack of significant improvement in this score may be because participants did not have access to the job search resources discussed in training, such as the Internet, once the program ended.

IMPLICATIONS AND FUTURE RESEARCH

While the findings of this study indicate that at-risk individuals' career search efficacy can be effectively enhanced by training that incorporates self-efficacy experiences, it is important to point out several limitations with our evaluation. For instance, the sample tested was rather small. The study also suffered from attrition as some participants voluntarily left the program and others were forced to leave due to attendance issues. In order to minimize these limitations in future research it is advisable that larger sample sizes be collected from various welfare-to-work training programs around the country. It also is important to point out that in the present study data were collected only twice. Pre-post measurement comparisons may not be sensitive enough to capture the process of change among long-term welfare recipients. Future research should measure career search efficacy several times throughout a program to more accurately assess if and how change(s) occur.

The current small sample size consisted of both welfare and non-welfare recipients. Solberg et al. (1994) acknowledged that career search efficacy research is important for improving the lives of individuals from many racial and ethnic minorities. Career search efficacy takes into account an individual's environment as a contributor toward change, thereby refocusing the beliefs of many individuals that their fate in life may be blamed solely on biases due to ethnicity. While all of the participants were from at-risk populations (i.e., the working poor), the OAI Community Kitchens training program provided an integrated environment in an effort to minimize the stigmatization associated with welfare recipients. Integrating both welfare and non-welfare groups in the current program may have attempted to break down barriers between social classes.

To improve personal exploration efficacy, job skill training for welfare recipients should actively engage participants to examine their professional goals and values from the start of the program. Trainers may want to point out how personal values often direct career values. In order to maintain improvements in career search efficacy, trainers also might provide participants with a variety of resources that are easy and readily available after training is completed.

REFERENCES

Bandura, A. (1986). The explanatory and predictive scope of self-efficacy theory. *Journal of Social and Clinical Psychology, 4*, 359-373.

Bandura, A. (1977). Self-efficacy: Toward a unifying theory of behavioral change. *Psychological Review, 84*, 191-215.

Chartrand, J.M., & Rose, M.L. (1996). Career interventions for at-risk populations: Incorporating social cognitive influences. *The Career Development Quarterly, 44*, 341-353.

Hackett, G., & Betz, N.E. (1981). A self-efficacy approach to the career development of women. *Journal of Vocational Behavior, 18*, 326-339.

Hughes, M., & Demo, D.H. (1989). Self-perceptions of Black Americans: Self-esteem and personal efficacy. *American Journal of Sociology, 95*, 132-157.

Pavetti, L. (1995) . . . And employment for all: Lessons from Utah's single parent employment demonstration project. Paper presented at the Seventeenth Annual Research Conference of the Association for Public Policy and Management, Washington, DC.

Solberg, V.S., Good, G.E., & Nord, D. (1994). Career search self-efficacy: Ripe for applications and intervention programming. *Journal of Career Development, 21*, 63-72.

Solberg, V.S., Good, G.E., Nord, D., Holm, C., Honer, R., Zima, N., Heffernan, M., & Malen, A. (1994). Assessing career search expectations: Development and validation of the Career Search Efficacy Scale. *Journal of Career Assessment, 2*, 111-123.

Sterrett, E.A. (1998). Use of job club to increase self-efficacy: A case study of return to work. *Journal of Employment Counseling, 35*, 69-78.

Swinton, D.H. (1992). The economic status of African Americans: Limited ownership and persistent inequality. In B.J. Tidwell (Ed.), *The State of Black America* (pp. 61-117). New York Urban League.

Welfare Reform and Women's Health: Challenges and Opportunities to Advance the Public Response to the Health Needs of Poor Women Through Monitoring and Collaboration

Lucia Rojas Smith
Patricia O'Campo
Holly Grason

Bloomberg School of Public Health

SUMMARY. The WCHPC studied the extent of collaboration between state women's health officials and TANF officials with respect to programs that affect the health and well-being of poor women. The kinds and extent of monitoring activities designed to gather information on the health status of this population were also examined. Great unevenness across states was revealed for both collaboration and monitoring. State-level interest in im-

---

Address correspondence to: Lucia Rojas Smith, RTI International, 1615 M Street NW, Washington, DC 20036 (E-mail: Lucia@rti.org).

Preparation of this manuscript was funded with grant #U93 MC 00101 from the Maternal and Child Health Bureau, Health Resources and Services Administration. The content does not necessarily reflect the views of the Bureau, HRSA, or the Department of Health and Human Services.

[Haworth co-indexing entry note]: "Welfare Reform and Women's Health: Challenges and Opportunities to Advance the Public Response to the Health Needs of Poor Women Through Monitoring and Collaboration." Rojas Smith, Lucia, Patricia O'Campo, and Holly Grason. Co-published simultaneously in *Journal of Prevention & Intervention in the Community* (The Haworth Press, Inc.) Vol. 23, No. 1/2, 2002, pp. 129-149; and: *The Transition from Welfare to Work: Processes, Challenges, and Outcomes* (ed: Sharon Telleen, and Judith V. Sayad) The Haworth Press, Inc., 2002, pp. 129-149. Single or multiple copies of this article are available for a fee from The Haworth Document Delivery Service [1-800-HAWORTH, 9:00 a.m. - 5:00 p.m. (EST). E-mail address: getinfo@haworthpressinc.com].

129

proving both was assessed, barriers to improvement were identified, and recommendations for steps forward were solicited. *[Article copies available for a fee from The Haworth Document Delivery Service: 1-800-HAWORTH. E-mail address: <getinfo@haworthpressinc.com> Website: <http://www. HaworthPress.com> © 2002 by The Haworth Press, Inc. All rights reserved.]*

KEYWORDS. Welfare reform, women's health, health monitoring, inter-agency cooperation

INTRODUCTION

In August 1996, the Personal Responsibility and Work Opportunity Reconciliation Act (P.L. 104-193; PRWORA) was signed into law ending a 60-year federal entitlement guaranteeing families a basic level of assistance during periods of economic hardship. Evaluations and policy studies examining the impact of welfare reform, as implemented through the program known as Temporary Assistance for Needy Families (TANF), thus far have focused almost exclusively on economic and child health outcomes (Acs & Pavetti, 1997; Connolly, 2000; Haskins, Sawhill & Weaver, 2001; Loprest, 1999; Chapin Hall Center, 2000; Cherlin et al., 2001). The impact of welfare reform on women's health, a potentially important factor in achieving full economic self-sufficiency, has been a minor consideration in research studies with the exception of access to health insurance (Callahan, 1999; Chavkin, Romero & Wise, 2000; Danziger et al., 1999; Garret & Holahan, 2000; Kneipp, 2000; Kramer, 2001; Winn & Lennon, 2000). Several aspects of the PRWORA have the potential to impact the health and well-being of women. These issues highlight areas of need and opportunity for state MCH Programs, offices on women's health, and welfare agencies to initiate new and/or strengthen current efforts on behalf of women and their families.

As a component of its work with the federal Maternal and Child Health Bureau to assist states in this regard, the Women's and Children's Health Policy Center (WCHPC) at the Johns Hopkins University Bloomberg School of Public Health undertook two related activities beginning in 1997. The first activity involved an extensive literature review examining the relationship between welfare, employment and health status (physical and mental), domestic violence, and access to health insurance. The findings from the literature review form the basis of a policy framework for monitoring the impact of welfare reform on women's health and well-being (O'Campo & Rojas Smith, 1998). These findings also provide the basis for articulating a set of strategies that states might pursue relative to protecting women's health interests under welfare reform. The second component of the WCHPC's work in this regard involved interviews with state and regional women's health and welfare officials. In these discussions, which took place between April 1999 and June 2000, the WCHPC sought to better understand selected aspects of activities in states concerning the health impacts of welfare reform for women.

This article summarizes key results of the *state interviews* and highlights potential venues through which state program directors and policymakers concerned with women's health and well-being might collaborate to advance public response to their needs.

Evidence from the literature review suggests that welfare reform can affect women's health in several ways. On the positive side, employment is associated with better psychological health, although these effects are not uniform for all types of employment. Low-wage, low-control jobs with little opportunity for personal input and self-development are associated with poor mental health outcomes (e.g., higher levels of depression, stress, and lower self-esteem). Other findings show that domestic violence, poor health (chronic conditions, mental health conditions) and need for health insurance are significant barriers to leaving welfare and maintaining stable employment.

In addition, certain groups of women are particularly vulnerable. For example, poor immigrant women, particularly those who entered the United States after August 1996, are no longer eligible for most Medicaid services. Moreover, vigilance is needed to ensure that appropriate public health prevention measures are in place in order to avoid increases in communicable disease rates among adolescents. States therefore need to devise strategies to otherwise ensure access to health care for these women, regardless of pregnancy status, in order to protect both individual and population health.

Changes in welfare instituted by PRWORA require poor women to enter the work force. Findings from the literature review suggest these jobs are low-wage positions with few or no health benefits. In addition, many beneficiaries of the TANF program are offered few opportunities for training or educational advancement and, thus, it is unclear whether over the long-term these women will be able to work themselves and their families out of poverty. Findings from the Urban Institute indicate that while women who have left welfare since PRWORA was enacted are marginally better off in terms of earnings compared to their working poor counterparts, they have not made substantive economic progress. One-third continue to experience difficulty providing sufficient food and shelter for their families.

Because welfare reform has the potential to affect women's health, monitoring and tracking the health and well-being of adult female TANF clients can provide important information about the links between welfare reform and women's health. The WCHPC therefore conducted a series of brief telephone interviews with regional and state level women's health and TANF officials to examine more fully the status of relevant monitoring activities. The goals of these interviews were to:

1. assess activities, currently underway in the states, designed to monitor the health and well-being of female TANF clients (current and former);
2. assess the interest among state officials in monitoring the health and well-being of female TANF clients (current and former) or in improving current monitoring efforts;
3. assess levels of collaboration and information sharing between women's health officials and TANF officials; and
4. raise awareness about the implications of welfare reform on women's health and well-being among state public health and human service program leaders and other policymakers.

METHOD

Interview participants came from two sources: the Office on Women's Health within the Department of Health and Human Services (DHHS), and TANF program officials identified by the Administration for Children and Families (ACF). Both sources included designated personnel for each of the 10 Regional Offices of the relevant federal agency and for each state including the District of Columbia.

Potential interviewees provided by the Office on Women's Health came from both state and federal appointments. A women's health contact is appointed by each state's public health commissioner and serves as a contact with the Office on Women's Health. This role is loosely defined; generally the contacts work to promote women's health issues within their state, and do this as part of, or in addition to, other duties of their position. Most of these individuals function within the maternal and child health or reproductive health units of their health departments, although a few are positioned within a chronic disease, primary care or women's health office. At the federal level, regional women's health coordinators are staff members of DHHS. Their role is solely dedicated to assisting the states in their region to promote awareness of and address women's health issues. They also serve as liaisons between the states and the federal Office on Women's Health. The coordinators meet on a periodic basis both within their region and in Washington, D.C. in order to share information, exchange ideas and promote initiatives addressing issues of concern to women's health. (Though they were part of the larger study, material from the 10 Regional Offices has not been included in this article.)

The Administration for Children and Families (ACF) has a similar network of state and regional TANF contacts. The Regional TANF Administrators are primarily responsible for assisting the states in their region to comply with federal mandates and address implementation issues and concerns. The State TANF contacts serve solely as point of contact for the ACF; they do not as a group meet routinely with either the regional TANF contact or federal ACF staff. Typically they are the commissioners or directors of the human services agencies responsible for TANF within their states. Our first communication with the TANF agency in each state was through these contacts, and in most cases we were referred to other personnel within the agency (i.e., TANF program managers) who had been appointed for an interview.

From April, 1999 to June, 2000 a total of 62 State Women's Health Contacts (n = 36) and TANF officials (n = 26) were interviewed by telephone. Participation was arranged through an introductory letter followed up by two to three phone calls, and in some cases a final faxed letter. Typically only one person was interviewed but in some cases additional colleagues were identified by the primary contact and included in the discussions. Forty-four states, including the District of Columbia, were represented in the sample in some way. The WCHPC was unable to obtain interviews from contacts in Massachusetts, Missouri, Oklahoma, Pennsylvania, South Dakota, Wisconsin, or Wyoming. Interviews were designed to last no more than 45 minutes; in some cases, depending on the informant's familiarity with the topics, they were much shorter.

In addition to the interviews, in order to provide additional background and contextual information, the study also reviewed state evaluations of welfare reform provided to the WCHPC by the respondents and evaluations posted on the website of the Research Forum on Children, Families and New Federalism. (Sponsored by the National

Center for Children in Poverty at Columbia University, this website reviews and lists all evaluations conducted at the state and federal levels to assess the impact of welfare reform, and is available at: http://www. researchforum.org.)

The interview guide developed for the state women's health contacts was composed entirely of open-ended questions that focused on four areas: (1) their perceptions of how welfare reform was affecting the health and well-being of poor women, adolescent women, immigrant women, and women facing domestic violence; (2) the types of monitoring activities (e.g., health insurance, health status, and domestic violence) taking place in their region; and (3) the extent of the informants' and their agency's involvement in, knowledge about, and perceptions of welfare reform issues.

In addition, a scale was developed to measure an informant's perceptions of each state's capacity to implement a comprehensive monitoring system, together with the level of collaboration between women's health and TANF officials at the state and federal levels.

Finally, recommendations were solicited for ways to heighten awareness of women's health monitoring in the context of welfare reform.

Because the term "health and well-being" covers an extraordinarily broad range of issues, we limited our analysis to monitoring activities related to: economic well-being (employment, wages); adolescent outcomes (education, employment and fertility); health insurance status; social support benefits (food stamps, child care and others); TANF diversionary program strategies; health barriers to work (chronic physical health problems and disabilities, mental health conditions, substance abuse); domestic violence; and family planning. For those respondents with high concentrations of immigrants we also asked about the effect of welfare reform on immigrant women's access to health care.

The term "monitoring" is defined to include any activity undertaken on a routine or periodic basis to collect and track information for the purposes of evaluation, program planning or program management. These included data gathering activities carried out by any state agency or independent contractor for the purpose of preparing routine reports, special studies, and short- and long-term outcome evaluations. With respect to health barriers and domestic violence, monitoring activities also included screening and follow-up treatment protocols. We did not consider information obtained solely through self-disclosure by the client to constitute monitoring (e.g., a client revealing unsolicited information about a health problem to a case worker), although information obtained through a client survey (a form of self-disclosure) was considered a monitoring activity. The interview guides were developed in a sequential and iterative manner such that the responses from one set of responses informed the content of the next set of interviews. In addition, being aware beforehand that not all categories of informants would be equally knowledgeable about monitoring activities, interviews were tailored to reflect this variability.

Interviews with State TANF contacts contained most of the elements used for the state women's health officials and added one additional item. For those states with decentralized programs administered by the county, we asked how decentralization affected uniform data collection.

RESULTS

Challenges and Opportunities for Interagency Collaboration

Since the successful implementation of welfare reform involves creating a host of partnerships including labor, employment, education, and health, to name a few, it has been suggested that collaboration between women's health officials and TANF officials should be an important area of consideration. The interviews revealed an overall unevenness in collaborative activities (see Table 1). This is based, apparently at least in part, on the differential degree of familiarity among this group of women's health and TANF interviewees with welfare populations and the programs offered to them.

Perhaps understandably, knowledge about welfare populations and programs was more limited on the part of the public health agency representatives interviewed. For example, interviews revealed that approximately one-half of the state women's health contacts did not have any information about whether or how health insurance status or health barriers of TANF program participants were monitored in their state. While nearly all the state women's health contacts we interviewed had some knowledge of domestic violence issues, many were not aware of how domestic violence was addressed for TANF clients.

The interviews did find that interagency collaboration was fairly routine at the regional level. However, a high degree of collaboration or partnering between public health and human services agencies responsible for TANF was not reflected in interviews with State Women's Health Contacts (mean reported collaboration = 2.8). The State Women's Health Contacts perceived interagency collaboration to be greater for their agency as a whole than for the specific office in which they were

TABLE 1. Cross-Agency Welfare Reform Activities

Activity	State Women's Health Contact	TANF
	n = 36 % (n)	n = 25 % (n)
serving on welfare reform planning group	31% (11)	20% (5)
implementing abstinence/fp programs	36% (13)	36% (9)
cross training staff/caseworkers	11% (4)	0
health department	n/a	20% (5)
domestic violence	5% (2)	44% (11)
mental health/substance abuse	0	12% (3)
Medicaid	16% (6)	28% (7)
employment/labor department	0	32% (8)

located. Again, this lower collaboration rating may have been due to less familiarity with issues regarding welfare reform.

Women's health respondents were asked to explain why they gave the ratings they did to their office or agency's level of involvement in welfare reform and interagency collaboration. A few themes emerged, although within a wide range of responses. Nearly one-third of the State Women's Health Contacts noted constraints on their involvement in welfare reform because of staff shortages, time limitations, or because the focus of their position did not include welfare reform (n = 10.) Overall, eight state women's health contacts expressed an interest in becoming more informed or involved in welfare reform issues, particularly with respect to monitoring the impact of welfare reform on women's health. A few, nonetheless, indicated that barriers in this regard were related to "agency turfism" (n = 3).

Among those women's health informants who believed interagency collaboration around welfare reform issues was good (a rating of 4 or 5), the most frequently cited reason was a positive environment of information exchange and sharing within their agency. Other reasons mentioned were statewide, multi-agency initiatives and proactive leadership among division and agency supervisors. These collaborations were most frequently related to welfare reform task forces, abstinence education for adolescents, and family planning programs for TANF clients. Other areas of collaboration included the cross-training of TANF case managers and eligibility workers, and providing Medicaid access for TANF clients. Although domestic violence is an area in which women's health officials reported involvement, only two were actively coordinating with TANF staff on these issues.

State TANF informants perceived a greater degree of interagency collaboration than did the respondents who discussed women's health (Mean rating of 4.1 vs. 2.8). Many noted that they generally worked with or communicated regularly with external programs and agencies, and they perceived it as an essential component of their work. The area with the highest degree of reported interagency collaboration was domestic violence. Most of this collaboration, though, was with local domestic violence shelters and not through a public health agency or unit in their state. Other than domestic violence, few TANF informants said that they or their staff work or communicate with women's health colleagues unless they needed to address abstinence policies, family planning, or Medicaid. A moderate level of involvement with other public health officials was reported, usually local health departments, on issues related to child health and other safety net services.

What States Reported About Monitoring Efforts

Just as interviews revealed an unevenness in the extent of collaborations between state women's health officials and TANF officials, a similar unevenness was discovered to be the case when it came to the variety of monitoring activities that could potentially be undertaken to gather information concerning the health and well-being of poor women. (See Table 2.)

Economic Well-Being

Monitoring the economic well-being of clients was an issue of great concern to informants at the state level. Nearly all the states participating in the interviews reported that some system was in place to track the employment status and wages of current TANF recipients. This was probably because all states were required by PRWORA to report this information on a routine basis to the U. S. Department of Health and Human Services. The level of sophistication in tracking economic indicators, however, varied substantially from state to state. Eight of the states reported the capacity to routinely track the employment and wages of former clients through well-integrated statewide labor data systems, through studies of former TANF clients (known as "leavers studies"), or a combination of both. A few states also had data sharing agreements with bordering states that allow them to track clients who leave their

TABLE 2. State Reports About Monitoring Selected Aspects of Women's Health (n = 44)

Kind of Report	Yes	Don't Know	No
Employment Wages	38		
Adolescent Pregnancy	10	2	14
Insurance	33	10	1
Benefits	35	8	1
Disability	16	27	1
Substance Abuse	28	14	1
Mental Health	20	21	3
Domestic Violence	19	21	4
Family Planning	1	5	19

state. A number of states (n = 11 in this study), however, did not have these types of information systems or arrangements, and relied primarily on leavers studies to periodically monitor economic indicators. Nine of the participating states reported undertaking extensive longitudinal studies of former clients (extending two or more years after leaving TANF).

Much of the public health policy emanating from PRWORA focused on adolescents in the form of pregnancy prevention, abstinence education, and requirements to live in an adult-supervised setting. In our sample, eight states undertook efforts to monitor the social and economic outcomes (educational attainment, employment and fertility) of adolescent parents receiving TANF. Where it existed, these monitoring activities were conducted either as part of routine data collection and evaluations or through evaluations of special programs for parenting adolescents. Though most states reported having a capacity to identify adolescents within their databases, they did not routinely report data separately for adolescents. Some of the TANF informants noted that the proportion of adolescent clients was too small to warrant additional reporting.

Other Public Benefit Use

Over two-thirds of the states participating in the interviews monitored the receipt of other support services such as food stamps, child care subsidies, transportation subsidies, and other assistance to current and former welfare clients. As with other economic indicators, the sophistication of the monitoring activities reported varied widely. Some of the states reported having integrated databases for TANF, Food Stamps and other benefits as well as the ability to routinely assess receipt of these services. Others relied primarily on periodic surveys and evaluations to monitor publicly funded support services.

Health Insurance Status

Most TANF clients are eligible for Medicaid coverage while participating in the program, yet because most states have now delinked cash assistance from Medicaid the risk of becoming uninsured due to administrative errors is greater than before. Thus, monitoring health insurance status among current and former clients is a key concern. Thirty-three of the states interviewed reported collecting some type of information on the health insurance status of their current and/or former clients; approximately 12 do so on a routine basis. The others used periodic surveys and evaluations to monitor health insurance status.

In addition to asking key informants about monitoring activities, discussions also touched on activities states have undertaken to inform women about their eligibility for Medicaid and other benefits once they leave TANF. Twelve states reported having implemented public information campaigns, distributing brochures, and/or sending letters to former TANF clients. Four of the states participating in WCHPC interviews reported that automatic redetermination systems were in place to ensure that women would not be automatically dropped from the Medicaid program once they left TANF. Four other states reported problems enrolling former clients in Medicaid. In these cases, the state was either not able to make contact with the former clients, and/or Medicaid coverage was mistakenly terminated even though the former client was still eligible for transitional coverage.

Three of the states in our sample had conducted statewide women's health surveys to gather data on health status and health insurance coverage. Other states indicated that they used the Behavioral Risk Factor Survey to gather similar information. One state was planning to implement a statewide survey of health insurance status. Only one of these states, however, had the capacity to identify TANF recipients within their sample or to provide reliable estimates for this population.

Health Barriers to Work

Chronic Conditions and Physical Disabilities. Federal reporting requirements mandate that all states report the number of clients exempted from work activities due to a physical disability. Beyond this basic level of tracking, however, reported monitoring of physical health barriers was uniformly limited. Most of our informants indicated that they collected only the information needed to keep track of the number of exemptions. None of the states interviewed reported having an assessment protocol in place to screen for latent physical disabilities that might potentially affect the type and duration of work activity. Only two states reported any special efforts to assist persons with disabilities to obtain work. A few, however, included physical disabilities in their outcome evaluations either as a descriptor or as one of a list of reasons for losing a job or returning to TANF (n = 3).

Substance Use. According to our interviews, of all the health barriers, substance use received the most attention. Over one-half of the states (n = 28) reported the existence of some type of system to address substance abuse, although the types of monitoring activities varied widely. Ten of these states noted having either a formal screening tool or a specialist contracted to counsel and assist substance using clients. A few states told us they assessed substance abuse mainly through self-disclosure. Other sources, however, indicated that 42 states use this form of detection (National Center on Addiction and Substance Abuse, 1999). Approximately 10 states also reported having a system in place to monitor the receipt of treatment services, although they did not necessarily have a formal assessment protocol. Where tracking of treatment did *not* occur, the respondents noted that confidentiality concerns prevented them from obtaining detailed information from substance abuse treatment facilities. In some states, tracking of treatment occurred through TANF contracts that stipulated treatment as a condition of receiving cash assistance, or treatment was considered an acceptable substitute for work activity.

Mental Health Conditions. Twenty of the states in our sample reported that they monitored mental health conditions either through a screening tool or a contracted mental health professional. Only about half of these states reported the ability to monitor the receipt of services due to the confidentiality reasons previously mentioned. Our review of the state evaluations of TANF programs showed that only two states examined mental health outcomes (e.g., depression, stress, etc.).

Domestic Violence. Nearly half of the 36 states for which we were able to obtain information on this topic reported monitoring domestic violence to some degree. However, about half of these states relied primarily on interviews by intake workers, and their competency to probe such sensitive issues was reported to vary widely. Only a handful of the states in our sample (n = 7) used a formal screening tool or domestic violence counselor to conduct assessments. Few states reported monitoring whether the client had received necessary services (n = 3). A number of the State Women's Health Contacts pointed out that even though their states had screening protocols in place, TANF clients were not being counseled and linked to services. Nine states reported having conducted special studies or otherwise examined in their evaluations domestic violence as a barrier to employment.

Family Planning. Although family planning has received a great deal of attention with respect to welfare reform via adolescent pregnancy prevention and bonuses provided to states for reducing out-of-wedlock birth rates, very little in the way of monitoring was reported. Only one state indicated routine assessment of the family planning needs of all female clients at intake, provision of counseling on site, and tracking of referrals. A small number of states indicated that they counseled clients about family planning services; however, these were reported to be relatively informal arrangements with no system in place to ensure the counseling was done on a routine basis. A small number of states reported using TANF block grant funds to purchase contraceptives for clients, while others reported using these funds to support abstinence education and shore up otherwise limited resources for other public family planning services.

Reported Interest in and Capacity for Monitoring Women's Health

In order to gain a greater appreciation for the status of welfare reform monitoring activities, the WCHPC investigators sought to learn about states' interest and capacity for monitoring as perceived by the informants. We asked the state women's health and TANF informants to rate, on a scale of one to five, the level of interest within their state in long-term monitoring of: (1) economic welfare of current and former TANF clients; (2) poor women's access to health insurance; (3) domestic violence among TANF clients; (4) measures of poor women's physical and mental health; and (5) occupational health hazards among women working in the low-wage sector.

The State Women's Health Contacts rated all items lower than did the TANF informants and were less sure of what the level of state interest was overall–ranging in all areas between 3.2 and 3.6. Nearly a fifth did not know or did not feel comfortable giving a rating for economic welfare or domestic violence. The TANF program ratings of interest with respect to these five areas were notably higher–ranging between 3.9 and 4.6. The TANF informants rated interest in economic welfare most highly, which could be expected given the focus on economic indicators in reporting requirements and evaluation studies. Similarly, the TANF contacts assigned their lowest rating to physical and mental health. Their ratings, however, reflected a higher level of interest than that of the women's health informants. It was unclear whether the higher ratings by the TANF informants conveyed a higher level of interest, or perhaps primarily a greater awareness of the activities underway.

With respect to assessment of a state's capacity to implement a comprehensive monitoring system that included the items in the scales, ratings were notably lower than those given for interest–again, an expected finding given that *interest* in monitoring does not necessarily correlate with *capacity* to monitor. TANF informants, however, did rate capacity higher than the women's health informants, which again may have to do with their different exposures to the issue, or to the relevance of data collection to the functions of their office.

Three barriers were cited repeatedly in response to questions about the most significant challenges to building an infrastructure for monitoring: (1) data integration; (2) data sharing; and (3) lack of interest. Many of the states reported grappling with how to link and interface data systems, particularly given limited fiscal and human resources available to devote to such tasks. Several states indicated that they were in the midst of implementing "new and improved" information systems and had encountered the need to invest heavily in worker retraining. Disruptions in the routine flow of reports and statistics needed for daily management of programs and contracts also were reported in a number of these instances.

Other informants believed their states had adequate information but that problems arose in the dissemination of that information. A number of informants expressed frustration with the many administrative obstacles they confronted in obtaining data about TANF clients in preparation for their interview. Better coordination and accessibility of existing data for them was the most important step towards building a better infrastructure through a central data warehouse and web-based access system. A common barrier cited was the lack of interest or leadership necessary to develop an integrated information system.

Another issue that was of particular concern in monitoring substance abuse, mental health and domestic violence was the need to protect the client's confidentiality. In this regard, a number of informants reported difficulty establishing collaborative partnerships with mental health and substance abuse agencies; thus they have been unable to collectively address the issues of confidentiality and monitoring. Informants from states that had some success in developing their information infrastructure were asked to tell us how their states had achieved those successes. Integrated eligibility databases for Medicaid, food stamps, child care and other support services were repeatedly cited as a key aid in coordinating monitoring and tracking activities. A few states had either received external funding or were planning to use their TANF surplus to upgrade their information systems. In one case, a state had used the mandated federal reporting requirements as political leverage to obtain additional state appropriations to upgrade their information systems.

Reported Challenges to and Opportunities for Monitoring Health Impacts of Welfare Reform on Women

Barriers to Monitoring

We asked the informants how the interest and capacity for women's health monitoring could be improved and a number of key barriers emerged: (1) limited awareness of the issues among political and/or administrative leaders; (2) limited political support for monitoring; and (3) limited attention to data coordination and distribution problems. At least a third of all of our interview participants felt that greater interest and political will among top administrators and legislators were needed to acquire the resources for a comprehensive monitoring of women's health indicators. Moreover, a few of the individuals with whom we spoke acknowledged that funding requests for monitoring might not be well-received because of political concerns about potentially uncovering problems and issues that might cost the state even more money. Better monitoring of women's health, they believed, could occur only if there was a public mandate to hold public officials accountable for welfare reform. Moreover, some of the women's health informants suggested that the prominence of women's health issues generally would have to be heightened among state administrators and political leaders before monitoring could be addressed within the context of welfare reform.

The TANF informants noted a number of barriers to evaluating the impact of welfare; foremost among these was the difficulty in tracking clients after they left the TANF program either because they had moved or the clients simply wanted no further contact with the TANF staff. One TANF informant, however, indicated success in contacting former clients (over 90%) for their leavers study, due primarily to the persistence of their field staff.

Another issue cited by numerous informants was the problem of accessing client data. Because many services for TANF clients were subcontracted, collecting and integrating data from these providers was difficult. Sharing data with mental health and substance abuse providers was especially difficult due to the concerns regarding confidentiality noted previously. A number of the informants talked of moving to a web-based system that would allow providers and TANF staff to input and download client data in a more efficient and coordinated fashion.

Inadequate capacity to evaluate programs and the need to build and develop local capacity to conduct welfare reform evaluations were also mentioned as concerns. In one state, the decision was made to hire local researchers with limited experience in welfare reform to conduct the TANF evaluation instead of an outside group of experts. The state's decision to invest in local capacity proved to be a prudent one. While there was an initial methodological learning curve to overcome, the local research group's knowledge of the culture and politics of their state added value to the evaluation. Moreover, their newly acquired expertise provided TANF administrators with a long-term asset that could be called upon for future studies and evaluations.

A few TANF informants whose states had used external consultants raised concerns. One noted difficulties encountered with their evaluators in developing a feasible study design given the state's small population size. A similar disregard for the limitations of the local environment was voiced by another informant. These reports suggested that while external consultants were well versed in statistical methodologies and study design overall, they and their clients had difficulty adapting rigorous research methods to practical circumstances.

A small number of the TANF informants believed their states relied too heavily on periodic, "one-shot" studies that quickly became outdated and forgotten. They hoped their states would develop a more institutionalized monitoring system that would provide routine analysis and estimates of key indicators of well-being. Such a system, they told us, would allow them to track their progress over time and be a useful tool for managing and developing programs suited to the needs of the client.

An issue discussed by a TANF informant that pertained to states with county-administered programs was the issue of state versus local control for monitoring and evaluation activities. Data for TANF programs that were state administered were centrally coordinated and thus generally more uniform. Moreover, state administrators determined what and how data should be collected and distributed. For county-administered programs, however, the locus of control for data collection was much more widely dispersed and state administrators might have little control over how monitoring was conducted. Developing a uniform monitoring system thus entailed significantly greater negotiation among many more players. In one county-administered state we surveyed, this issue had been successfully addressed and a uniform data collection system implemented. Another state, however, resorted to legal action to prompt a number of their counties to comply with federal reporting requirements.

Factors Enabling Improved Monitoring

In addition to discussing the barriers to monitoring, we encouraged those we interviewed to tell us what types of policies, resources and other assistance would help improve the monitoring of women's health in their state. Their responses were varied, but TANF and women's health informants both emphasized the need for fiscal and human resources to upgrade and integrate information systems. One individual suggested that the federal government develop a national employment database to help track clients who move from state to state. Some of the informants indicated the need for agency staff assigned exclusively to evaluation and research functions and the development of better indicators/measures of performance.

A less prominent but important finding that emerged from this portion of the interviews dealt with the role of the federal government. While a very small number of informants believed the federal reporting requirements to be cumbersome and unreasonable, a few informants welcomed a stronger federal presence. In two states, the federal reporting mandates had been helpful not only in the identification of key indicators but in securing additional resources for system upgrades. In another state, a federal audit of the Medicaid program had provided the external pressure necessary to compel the state legislature to address inadequacies in the system. The informants from this state believed that an audit of the TANF program could be similarly instrumental. These responses indicated that despite the rhetoric of "local control," program administrators may feel powerless to address important but unpopular issues due to the constraints of their political environment. These cases suggested that a greater federal role either in the form of mandates, audits or technical assistance could be helpful and constructive in these situations.

DISCUSSION

The monitoring of welfare reform and women's health has received little attention among policymakers, but it presents numerous opportunities for communication and collaboration across disciplines and agencies. Our interviews with women's health and TANF informants indicated that economic welfare, other public benefit use, health insurance and substance abuse were the most closely monitored indicators of women's health and well-being. However, the breadth and scope of this monitoring was reported to vary substantially. Domestic violence and mental health conditions were less closely monitored but still received at least moderate levels of attention among those states for which we were able to obtain information. Physical disabilities and family planning were reported to be the least closely monitored. Almost none of the states we interviewed had a substantive system in place to monitor these health conditions or included them in their evaluations. Overall, our TANF informants believed their state would be interested in monitoring women's health and well-being. The state women's health contacts rated state interest in monitoring more moderately. In general, our informants rated their state capacity for monitoring lower than their interest, although the state TANF informants gave higher ratings than the State Women's Health Contacts.

Our women's health informants were as a group less familiar with welfare reform issues and were less involved in activities that entailed interacting with TANF colleagues. Of those who did collaborate with TANF colleagues, most were involved in projects related to abstinence education, family planning services and/or cross-training of TANF case-workers on these and other health programs. Domestic violence was reported to be a high priority issue for many of the women's informants but very few were working with TANF colleagues on this issue.

Our informants cited numerous barriers to monitoring women's health; foremost among these was a lack of interest among program administrators and legislators. Many of the informants indicated that generating greater political will would be an essential prerequisite to address another frequently mentioned barrier, inadequate information systems. Data issues featured prominently in our discussions, with many of our informants including challenges to developing new information systems, retraining workers to new systems, and disseminating available information in a timely and efficient manner.

A number of issues related to evaluation capacity also emerged from our interviews including the need for more resources devoted exclusively to such activity, the challenges of building up local capacity, and working with external evaluators to develop feasible study designs. Confidentiality was repeatedly mentioned as a concern among those we interviewed. Many noted this was a key issue in monitoring substance abuse, mental illness, and domestic violence. Thus, while at least half or more of the states for which we were able to obtain information routinely screened for these conditions, few states reported developing a system for ensuring women received needed services, or that these services were of a high quality.

Beyond the barriers identified, one interesting and noteworthy enabling factor emerged from our interviews. In a few of the states, a constructive federal presence had facilitated better monitoring either through helping to secure additional state appropriations for evaluations or helping evaluators to develop a set of core indicators for a new monitoring system.

The discussions with women's health and TANF informants highlighted a number of opportunities to improve the monitoring of the health and well-being of current and former participants in the TANF program. While the WCHPC interviews and this article focus specifically on Office on Women's Health (OWH) and ACF professionals involved with women's health, our findings point also to the relevant and important roles that state Title V Maternal and Children Health programs can play in strategies to address concerns identified in this brief. State Maternal and Child Health (MCH) programs can offer specific expertise related to a number of women's health issues that surfaced from the interviews, but especially in areas such as data and information on women's health and health status, strategies and tools for clinical screening of women regarding their risk status for health conditions relevant to welfare reform (e.g., substance abuse, contraceptive use), and referral and tracking of women who require specialized services and care.

In light of these findings, we hope that states will consider pursuing the following strategies to further ensure greater appreciation for and commitment to addressing the effects that welfare reform may have on the woman's total well-being.

1. *Continue to build awareness of the broad spectrum of women's health concerns, and incorporate welfare reform as part of the women's health agenda.*

The implications of welfare reform on women's health could be more readily understood if women's health professionals and advocates at both the state and regional levels were kept abreast of welfare reform policy. Similarly, systems enhancements might arise if welfare officials had a better understanding of women's health. Sponsoring joint educational conferences and policy forums might facilitate this awareness. Greater efforts also could be given to dissemination of relevant data reports and study findings.

2. Increase awareness of the need for better monitoring of women's health generally, and in specific regard to women participating in welfare programs. Increase collaborative efforts for this monitoring.

The monitoring of welfare reform is a cross-cutting endeavor that has the potential to bring together various agencies responsible for the health and social services needs of poor women. Abstinence education, family planning, access to Medicaid and other health insurance, and domestic violence are all areas of mutual concern to women's health, TANF, and Title V MCH professionals. Discussions regarding how these issues can best be monitored could serve as a fertile ground for unique and constructive partnerships among these groups.

For instance, while there appears to be concerted efforts in some states to monitor economic well-being, public benefit use and health insurance status, more attention is needed in the areas of physical disabilities, mental health, substance abuse, domestic violence and family planning. In this particular regard, state Title V MCH programs might be called upon as partners in identifying existing and/or developing new screening and assessment instruments and to confer with welfare officials about referral resources and protocols.

Additionally, as noted by a number of those interviewed by the WCHPC, a federal role in this regard may be important, and valued by the states. Consideration might profitably be given to a federal-regional-state effort among women's health, TANF, and Title V (and others, such as SAMHSA, OPA, HCFA, etc.) to develop national indicators, and provide technical assistance for states.

REFERENCES

Acs, G., & Pavetti, L. (1997, July). *Study of the employment patterns of young women and the implication for welfare mothers: How much more can they work? Setting realistic expectations for welfare mothers* (Assessing the New Federalism Policy Analysis Project). Washington, DC: Urban Institute.

Callahan, S. (1999). *Understanding health status barriers that hinder the transition from welfare to work.* Washington, DC: National Governor's Association.

Chapin Hall Center for Children (2000, January). *Monitoring child and family social program outcomes: Before and after welfare reform in four states: Outcomes for the income maintenance caseload during receipt.* Chicago: University of Chicago Chapin Hall Center for Children.

Chavkin, W., Romero, D., & Wise, P.H. (2000). State welfare reform policies and declines in health insurance. *American Journal of Public Health. 90*, 6, 900-8.

Cherlin, A., Burton, B., Francis, J., Henrici, J., Lein, L., Quane, J., & Bogen, K. (2001, February). *Sanctions and case closings for noncompliance. Who is affected and why. Welfare, children and families: A three city study* (Policy Brief 01-1). Baltimore: The Johns Hopkins University.

Connolly, L.S. (2000, May). *The effect of welfare reform on the incomes and earning of low-income families: Evidence from the Current Population Survey.* Paper presented at the meeting, Rural Dimension of Welfare Reform: A Research Conference on Poverty, Welfare and Food Assistance, Washington, DC.

Danzinger, S., Corcoran, M., Heflin, D.M., Kalil, A., Levine, J., Rosen, D., Seefeldt, K., Siefert, K., & Tolman, R. (1999, May). *Barriers to the employment of welfare recipients* (Working Paper No. 90). Chicago: Joint Center for Poverty Research.

Garret, G., & Holahan, J. (2000, March). *Welfare leavers, medicaid coverage and private insurance* (Brief No.13, Assessing the New Federalism Policy Analysis Project). Washington, DC: Urban Institute.

Haskins, R., Sawhill, I., & Weaver, K. (2001, January). *Welfare reform: An overview of effects to date* (WR&B Policy Brief 1). Washington, DC: Brookings Institution.

Kneipp, S.M. (2000). The health of women in transition from welfare to employment. *Western Journal of Nursing Research, 6*, 656-74.

Kramer, F.D. (2001, February). Screening and assessment for physical and mental health issues that impact TANF recipients ability to work. *Issue Notes* [Online serial] 5, 3 (Welfare Information Network). Available http://www.welfareinfo.org.

Loprest, P. (1999). *How families that left welfare are doing: A national picture* (Brief Series B, No B-1, Assessing the New Federalism Policy Analysis Project). Washington, DC: Urban Institute.

National Center on Addiction and Substance Abuse (1999, August). *Building bridges: States respond to substance abuse and welfare reform.* New York: Columbia University.

O'Campo, P., & Rojas Smith, L. (1998). Welfare reform and women's health: Review of the literature and implication for state policy. *Journal of Public Health Policy, 19*, 4 (Winter), 420-446.

Winn, E., & Lennon, M.C. (2000, March). The role of administrative data and national data sets in understanding welfare reform. *The Forum* [Online serial], 3, 1 (Research Forum on Children, Families and the New Federalism). Available: http://www.researchforum.org.

The Effect of State Welfare Waivers on Family Earnings and Income Growth of AFDC Recipients, 1993-1995

Laura S. Connolly

University of Northern Colorado

SUMMARY. Many observers of welfare reform have argued that self-sufficiency on the part of welfare recipients is desirable. This would require, at least, that recipients' economic well-being not fall as a result of welfare reform. That question is addressed here by analyzing the impact of early state-level welfare waivers on the growth of earnings and income received by welfare recipients. Analysis of data from the Current Population Survey found that among welfare recipients (1) early work-related welfare reforms generally did not improve the growth in family earnings, and (2) waivers often had a small but negative effect on the growth of family income. Waivers were less detrimental for rural than for urban recipients. Since research has shown that rural employment and earnings generally lag behind urban areas, this is an interesting finding. It sug-

Address correspondence to: Laura S. Connolly, Department of Economics, Campus Box 101, Greeley, CO 80639 (E-mail: LSCONNO@unco.edu).

An abridged version of this article appears under the title "The Effect of Welfare Reform on the Incomes and Earnings of Low-Income Families: Evidence from the Current Population Survey" in *Confronting Poverty in the Wake of Welfare Reform* (2002), edited by Frances Fox Piven, Joan Acker, Margaret Hallock, and Sandra Morgen, Eugene OR: University of Oregon Press (2002).

[Haworth co-indexing entry note]: "The Effect of State Welfare Waivers on Family Earnings and Income Growth of AFDC Recipients, 1993-1995." Connolly, Laura S. Co-published simultaneously in *Journal of Prevention & Intervention in the Community* (The Haworth Press, Inc.) Vol. 23, No. 1/2, 2002, pp. 151-175; and: *The Transition from Welfare to Work: Processes, Challenges, and Outcomes* (ed: Sharon Telleen, and Judith V. Sayad) The Haworth Press, Inc., 2002, pp. 151-175. Single or multiple copies of this article are available for a fee from The Haworth Document Delivery Service [1-800-HAWORTH, 9:00 a.m. - 5:00 p.m. (EST). E-mail address: getinfo@haworthpressinc.com].

151

gests that even though rural residents face greater barriers to employment, welfare reform has a smaller marginal effect on rural recipients. *[Article copies available for a fee from The Haworth Document Delivery Service: 1-800-HAWORTH. E-mail address: <getinfo@haworthpressinc.com> Website: <http://www.HaworthPress.com> © 2002 by The Haworth Press, Inc. All rights reserved.]*

KEYWORDS. Current Populations Survey, synthetic panel, welfare reform, low-income women, income

INTRODUCTION

The Personal Responsibility and Work Opportunity Reconciliation Act of 1996 (PRWORA), federal legislation P.L. 104-193, dramatically restructured the way assistance is provided to needy families. Despite empirical evidence showing that much of the drop in welfare caseloads since then has resulted from the strong economy rather than welfare reform (Ziliak, Figlio, Davis, & Connolly, 2000; U.S. Council of Economic Advisers, 1997), many advocates of welfare reform have pointed to the dramatic drop in caseloads as evidence of the success of the newly designed programs. Recently, however, discussion has turned to the more difficult question of how former recipients are faring in the wake of welfare reform. Since the work requirements enacted under PRWORA are very similar to those adopted by many states prior to PRWORA, the experience of welfare recipients in states with these requirements is relevant to upcoming deliberations concerning the renewal of the current federal law. This paper examines the effect of early state-level welfare reform policies, those which took place prior to the adoption of PRWORA, on the growth in earnings and total income of those families who received Aid to Families with Dependent Children (AFDC) and other cash benefits when the reforms were enacted.

Recently a number of studies have been conducted in which former welfare recipients were interviewed at regular intervals (Brauner & Loprest, 1999). These provide valuable information but still yield an incomplete picture of the status of those who have left the welfare rolls. By design, they enhance our understanding of the situation in a specific geographical area under a specific set of policy and economic conditions, but are not easily generalized. In addition, the expense and difficulty of following former recipients in rural areas make it likely (but not inevitable) that the information revealed by this type of study will focus primarily on the effects in urban areas.

An alternative is to use longitudinal data from national surveys or administrative sources. The advantage of longitudinal data is the ability to follow the same recipient over a long period of time, thus documenting the dynamics of welfare use in addition to the short-term effects of welfare policy. This makes longitudinal studies extremely valuable. However, there are some disadvantages to most of these data sets as well. For example, the recipients included in the National Longitudinal Survey of Youth are relatively younger than the recipient population as a whole (Cancian et al., 1999). In addition, while most national longitudinal surveys have reasonably large sample sizes it is not always possible to examine the effects of policy changes on the population subsets of interest. Administrative data may contain a larger and more representative sample for a given state, but generally cannot be linked across states, so cannot as easily be used to generalize about welfare policy. In addition, administrative data from many states do not contain the wealth of demographic information contained in most national longitudinal data sets.

It is possible to both gain the advantages of longitudinal data sets and avoid some of their problems by creating a synthetic panel data set from the March supplements of the Current Population Survey (CPS). The main advantages of using the CPS are that it is a very large and nationally representative data set, it contains very detailed information on demographics and income sources, and it permits an examination of the effects of welfare reform on the family income and earnings growth of former recipients living in both urban and rural areas.

Specifically, the CPS data can be used to predict changes in family incomes and earnings over time, after which statistical analysis can be used to differentiate the effects of welfare reform and economic conditions on these changes. The specific focus is to determine whether welfare reform furthers one of the goals explicitly stated in PRWORA: "to end the dependence of needy parents on government benefits by promoting job preparation, work, and marriage" (Title I, sec. 401(a)(2)). If proponents of welfare reform are correct in their assumption that work is the key to self-sufficiency, then, holding other relevant variables constant, families who received public assistance and lived in states that enacted reforms with strict work requirements or increased work incentives should have higher income and earnings growth than their counterparts living in states without such reforms. However, if welfare reform is making it more difficult for families to make ends meet, then the opposite should occur. Use of CPS data makes it possible to test these sharply contrasting expectations by comparing the outcomes of such families in states that did and states that did not receive waivers.

METHOD

Conceptual Foundations for the Model

A four-way categorization of variations in state welfare policies can provide the basis for examining the effects of these variations on welfare recipients. State level policies enacted before PRWORA were allowed under waivers from the federal rules regulating AFDC. For this reason they are frequently referred to, and will be referred to here, simply as "waivers." The requirements and conditions imposed by these waivers varied substantially across states, and have been categorized in many ways (U.S. Council of Economic Advisers, 1997; Crouse, 1999; Ziliak et al., 1997, 2000). For the purposes of the present study, however, it is useful to group them into three categories: (1) *work requirements,* which require work (or participation in a job training or job search program) as a condition of eligibility to receive public assistance; (2) *work incentives,* which increase the economic value of work on the part of recipients (e.g., by increasing the earnings one can receive without losing AFDC benefits), and (3) *all other* provisions. This broad categorization makes it possible to focus on the effect of work-related waivers (work requirements and work incentives), both jointly and separately, on earnings and incomes. An additional category, provided as a comparison, examines the effect of all types of waivers combined.

The interaction of requirements and incentives may affect earnings and income in different ways. *Earnings* are that portion of an income that has been paid as compensation for work. Not all income must derive from work, however; just as the interest on a certificate of deposit is not classed as "earned income," neither is a cash benefit that derives from a person's participation in an entitlement program. Even though non-cash benefits are not considered income for the purposes of these studies, it is still the case that for many people a family's *total income* is a complex mix of earnings and other forms of income. Welfare reforms thus may have distinct effects on earnings and income.

Economic theory yields ambiguous predictions regarding the expected effect of work requirements on the earnings of welfare recipients (Ehrenberg & Smith, 1994). Some work requirement waivers took the form of "workfare," which required that the recipient work at a public job and be "paid" the welfare benefit in lieu of a wage. Because welfare benefits were not counted as earned income, in such cases measured earnings would not change in the short run. Similarly, there would be no immediate earnings or income effect for those who must participate in job search or job training activities instead of working at a publicly provided job. However, the assumption underlying many of the work requirements was that welfare recipients would move into higher paying, more stable jobs (and off the welfare rolls) once they had gained work experience or training. If so, then the earnings of these individuals would be expected to rise after some period of time.

Work incentives, which may or may not have been combined with work requirements, could also have ambiguous effects on earnings. In the original AFDC program the "30 and 1/3 rule" allowed the recipient to keep the first $30, plus 33%, of any wages earned during the first four months on AFDC. After the first four months benefits were reduced by one dollar for each dollar of earnings. Work incentive waivers allowed a recipient to keep at least a portion of her benefit in addition to her wages, rather than decreasing benefits dollar-for-dollar after the first four months. While this would generally be expected to increase work effort among recipients, it would only do so if the additional income outweighed the extra costs of working. These costs, which include child care, transportation, clothing, and, in many cases, health insurance, can be substantial and often were not covered by the increased benefits (Edin & Lein, 1997).

While it is important to determine the effect of waivers on earnings growth, it is perhaps even more critical to understand what happens to growth in total income. After all, a family's well-being derives from income from *all* sources, which for these families could include both earnings and welfare support. Since increased earnings led to decreased benefits, incomes would not necessarily rise with work effort. (Non-cash assistance was also reduced, which may also have eroded the value of increased earnings, but since this is not counted as income it will not be addressed here.) Blank (1997, ch. 3) and, especially, Tapogna and Witt (1998) have provided fascinating examples of the ways in which, at varying levels of work effort, the interactions among public assistance programs affect incomes.

Incomes could also be reduced for other reasons. In addition to work requirements and/or incentives, many waivers imposed sanctions for certain types of behaviors. Recipients who were unable to comply with these provisions found their benefits reduced, thereby reducing their incomes.

The Empirical Model

To empirically examine the question of whether work-related waivers cause earnings and incomes to grow more or less quickly than in states without such waivers it is first necessary to isolate the effect of these waivers from other factors that affect earnings and income growth. It is possible to do this using a two-step approach. First, earnings and income growth in states with waivers are compared to states having similar economic conditions but no waivers. This comparison provides the "difference" coefficient. It isolates the effect of waivers from the effect of economic conditions as well as unobservable factors that are similar in both waiver and non-waiver states.

The effect of waivers at the state level may, however, still be confounded with other unobservable factors that differ across states. Therefore the second step is to provide a "difference-in-difference" coefficient by comparing the waiver effects found for welfare recipients with those of two other categories of families used as control groups: (1) all non-recipient families, and (2) families headed by non-recipient single females. Though non-recipient families headed by single females may, because of their similarities with the group of recipients, appear to be better for comparison than all non-recipient families, families headed by single females are not suitable as a sole source of comparison because welfare reform may affect the behavior of single females who were not recipients at the time of the reform. For example, some of these women may have found welfare a more attractive option after a work incentive waiver is introduced. This would imply that their labor supply, and therefore their earnings, could *decrease* as a result. Similarly, a work requirement waiver that subsidized job training may have induced some non-recipients to apply for AFDC if they believed that this training would lead to a better job than they currently held. See Moffitt (1996) for a discussion of the incentive effects of these programs. For that reason both categories–all non-recipient families and those headed by single females–are used as control groups. Any changes in earnings and income growth that are due to factors other than waivers should be the same for both the control groups and the AFDC recipients, so any systematic difference between AFDC families and the control groups can be attributed to waivers.

Finally, previous literature has shown that the impact of policies directed at alleviating poverty is often dissimilar in urban and rural areas. This is due to differences in both labor force behavior and labor demand conditions in rural and urban areas (e.g., Deavers & Hoppe, 1992; Davis, Connolly, & Weber, 2001; Findeis & Jensen, 1998; Findeis et al., 1992). For this reason the sample has been separated into rural and urban residents and the analysis repeated. The U.S. Office of Management and Budget definition has been used to identify rural and urban families: Rural means not living in a Metropolitan Statistical Area (MSA), urban is the opposite. This is not a perfect indicator of whether a person lives in a rural area because the county in which she lives may be included in an MSA even if many parts of the county are sparsely populated. (Weber, Acock, and Goetz [1991] provide a thorough discussion of alternative definitions of "rural" and "urban.") The consequence of using the Office of Management and Budget designation of rural and urban areas is that, by treating all residents of MSAs as urban and everyone else as rural, the number of rural residents in the sample will be undercounted. Differences between the two types of residents will tend to be obscured, so any differences that are found provide a strong indication that actual differences are at least as large. If the difference-in-difference coefficients for urban residents are significantly different from those of rural families, then welfare reform has a differential impact in the two areas.

One problem with using the CPS for this analysis can be overcome by using methodology developed by Connolly and Segal (2001) to construct a longitudinal data set "synthetically." The CPS follows a given household for only one year so it cannot directly be used to observe long-term changes in family incomes or earnings. It is important to follow those families who were receiving cash assistance *before* welfare reform policies took effect, so it is not sufficient to examine the incomes and earnings of the set of families who are observed in the CPS in the years following the reforms. Instead, the analysis needs a data set that follows the same families over time (a "longitudinal" data set). A "synthetic panel" can do this. Several steps are involved. The first, using the March CPS survey containing data for post-reform years, is to estimate an income or earnings equation for those years. The second is to predict the post-reform income and earnings of families observed in the year immediately preceding reform by using their demographics and other relevant information in the estimated income and earnings equations). The estimation process (known to economists as "tobit estimation") accounts for the fact that income and (especially) earnings may be censored at zero. (Censoring at zero means that the true values might be negative, if that were possible, but since it is not the distribution of incomes and earnings is "cut off" [i.e., "censored"] at zero.) It also allows for correlation in the residuals of these equations across years (Moffitt & Gottschalk, 1995). The synthetic panel makes it possible to predict the change in family earnings and incomes that is used in the difference-in-difference analyses discussed previously.

Construction of the Synthetic Panel

The goal is to calculate the growth of family earnings and income between two points in time that are not necessarily consecutive. Since the CPS has limited data on these variables for the same family over time, the model used the family's actual earnings or income in the year in which they were observed and the predicted earnings and income in the second period. This set of two observations per family is the synthetic panel. For ease of exposition, the methodology is described in terms of family earnings. The process is identical for income estimation.

The first step is to predict each family's second period earnings. This is done by first estimating, using data on families actually observed during the second period, a model of the natural log of family earnings for that period.[1] The model estimates the effect on earnings of a variety of demographic variables and of the state in which the family resides. Demographic characteristics of the householder included in the model are gender, marital status, veteran status, race, age, and education (including quadratic terms in age and education). Family characteristics included are place of residence (urban, central city, or other), the number of children aged 18 or less, and the number of adults (male and female). Differences in economic conditions and other state-level characteristics are controlled for by a set of indicator variables for the state of residence.

Once a model has been created that estimates the effect of demographic variables and state characteristics on earnings during Period 2, this model can then be used to predict the second period earnings of the families observed in the base year (Year 1). This can be done because each of the two samples has been drawn from the same population using the same sampling methodology. (An implication is that the only difference between the estimated model and one based on actual Year 2 data for the base sample of families, were it available, is due to sampling variability.)

The model must also control for correlations among the year-to-year earnings of families over and above those accounted for by the factors used in the model. If the demographic and state-level variables included in the prediction equation perfectly captured all factors that could be expected to influence earnings, then the predicted log earnings for each family would be obtained by simply plugging the appropriate Period 1 demographic and state variables into the equation.[2] However, it is likely that there are additional unobserved family characteristics that influence earnings, meaning that the residuals for a given family are likely to be correlated across years. Research by Moffitt and Gottschalk (1995) suggests that this correlation is generally above 0.6. They estimate the correlation of the residuals from a log annual earnings equation for white males. Their estimates vary depending on the cohort, averaging 0.76 for the 1986-1987 time span. The correlation for this sample is likely to be higher because it considers family, rather than individual, earnings and incomes. For that reason 0.6 has been used as a lower bound when calculating the predicted earnings.

Finally, the estimate of the Period 2 predicted earnings may be negative, but observed earnings are not. In cases where the prediction is negative, zero has been used instead.

The predicted log income has been calculated in the same way. The synthetic panel consists of actual log earnings and log income in Year 1 and predicted log earnings and log income in Year 2.

Identification of the Welfare Reform Effect

To determine the effect of welfare reform, first the synthetic panel is used to compute the difference between the predicted Year 2 log earnings and the observed Year 1 log earnings for each family. The difference approximates the growth of earnings over the period. Next this variable is regressed on a variable defined by one of the four categories of state welfare waivers (discussed at the beginning of this section and in detail in the next section) and on two variables that control for differences in economic growth across states: (1) the change in the state unemployment rate between Year 1 and Year 2, and (2) the change in Gross State Product over the two years.[3]

The estimated effect of the waiver variable measures the percentage point difference in predicted earnings growth for a family who lives in a state with a waiver compared to an otherwise similar family living in a non-waiver state with the same level of economic growth. Because attention has not been restricted to families who were receiving welfare in Period 2, the effect on those who left the rolls is implicitly included.

DATA

Measures of Earnings, Income, and Demographics

Data on family earnings, incomes, and demographics are taken from several years of the March surveys of the Current Population Survey. The CPS is valuable for this type of study because it includes information on participation in a wide variety of public assistance programs, as well as detailed data on demographic characteristics and sources of income and earnings for a large, representative, sample of U.S. households. Indeed, Moffitt (1999) recently argued for the use of the CPS microdata for studying the effects of welfare reform on a variety of outcomes, including those examined here (earnings and incomes). Another important advantage of the CPS is that it provides information on family, not just individual, incomes and earnings. Welfare reform affects entire families, not just individuals, so it is important to determine how family level resources are affected.

Families were coded as (1) *recipients of public assistance*, in contrast to (2) *non-recipients*, if they answered "yes" to a question asking whether, at any time in the last year, any member of the household had received any public assistance from state or local sources. To use the CPS for studies such as this it is necessary that interviewees honestly report family participation in assistance programs. There is no evidence to suggest that participation levels are underreported in the CPS. There is some evidence that the *amount* of public assistance received is underreported in the CPS. This will cause measurement error in the income variable, but will not affect the dependent variable used here (the *change* in log incomes) unless underreporting is systematically different across years.

Measures of Welfare Reform

Many states received waivers from the standard federal regulations governing public assistance programs (especially AFDC) during the mid-1990s, allowing them to experiment with work requirements, time limits and a number of other policies. The model was estimated using four different definitions of the waiver variable: (1) *any work related* waiver, which combines all waivers that contain work requirements or provide additional incentives for work; (2) *work requirement* waivers only; (3) *work incentive* waivers only; and (4) *any* waiver, which combines waivers of any type, whether work-related or not.[4] The variables used here to measure welfare reform were based upon information available from the U.S. Department of Health and Human Services (Crouse, 1999). Many waivers covered only small portions of the caseload, e.g., a single county, but only waivers that applied statewide were used in this study.[5] Though states continued to receive waivers through most of 1996 (until the passage of PRWORA), this study examines only waivers implemented by the end of 1993 and 1994. For those waivers in effect for only part of a year, a variable was created that equals the fraction of the year for which a given state had a waiver in effect. For example, if a state implemented a waiver in October of 1993, then for that state this variable would equal 0 before 1993, 0.25 in 1993, and 1.0 thereafter.

RESULTS

Full Sample, Rural and Urban Residents Pooled

Table 1 presents the effect of welfare waivers on the earnings and income of all recipients and all non-recipients of public assistance, without regard for the gender, marital status, or rural versus urban residence of the householder. First, Table 1 shows the coefficient estimates on the welfare waiver variable for all four waiver conditions over the three time periods considered. The 1993-94 and 1993-95 time periods capture the one- and two-year effects, respectively, of waivers that were implemented before or during 1993. The 1994-95 period indicates the one-year effect of all waivers implemented by the end of 1994. The coefficients show the size of the difference made in the earnings and income of residents living in states with waivers compared with residents of non-waiver states. For example, the first estimate given in column 1, the difference coefficient for recipients of public assistance in 1993-94, would indicate that predicted earnings growth of a recipient living in a state with a work-related waiver was 0.038 percentage points lower than that of a similar recipient living in a non-waiver state, though this particular estimate is statistically insignificant. For example, if a recipient's earnings grew at five percent in the non-waiver state, then this es-

TABLE 1. Differential Effect of Welfare Waivers on Growth in the Earnings and Income of Recipients of Public Aid, by Time Period (Full Sample)

Aid Recipient Status	Earnings: change in predicted growth of earnings with respect to kind of waiver				Income: change in predicted growth of income with respect to kind of waiver			
	Any work-related (1)	Work require-ment (2)	Work Incentive (3)	Any waiver (4)	Any work-related (5)	Work require-ment (6)	Work Incentive (7)	Any waiver (8)
				1993-1994				
Recipient[a]								
coefficient	−0.038	−0.299**	0.109	−0.034	−0.072***	−0.040	−0.061***	−0.043***
(s.e.)	(0.067)	(0.116)	(0.085)	(0.060)	(0.016)	(0.027)	(0.020)	(0.014)
Non[a]								
coefficient	0.043***	−0.066***	0.089***	0.009	−0.004	−0.023**	0.005	−0.002
(s.e.)	(0.013)	(0.022)	(0.017)	(0.011)	(0.007)	(0.011)	(0.009)	(0.006)
Difference	−0.081	**−0.233**	0.020	−0.043	**−0.068***	−0.017	**−0.066***	**−0.041***
p-value	0.23	0.05	0.82	0.48	0.00	0.55	0.00	0.01
				1993-1995				
Recipient								
coefficient	−0.045	−0.219*	0.073	−0.063	−0.044***	−0.036	−0.033	−0.026*
(s.e.)	(0.070)	(0.121)	(0.090)	(0.062)	(0.017)	(0.029)	(0.022)	(0.015)
Non[a]								
coefficient	0.059***	0.032	0.060***	−0.018	0.030***	−0.009	0.038***	0.013**
(s.e.)	(0.013)	(0.022)	(0.017)	(0.011)	(0.007)	(0.011)	(0.009)	(0.006)
Difference	−0.104	**−0.251**	0.013	−0.045	**−0.074***	−0.027	**−0.071***	**−0.039**
p-value	0.15	0.04	0.88	0.48	0.00	0.39	0.00	0.02
				1994-1995				
Recipient [b]								
coefficient	0.127*	0.126	0.221**	0.060	−0.025	−0.005	−0.022	−0.019
(s.e.)	(0.069)	(0.122)	(0.103)	(0.060)	(0.018)	(0.032)	(0.027)	(0.016)
Non[b]								
coefficient	0.034***	0.142***	−0.021	−0.007	0.038***	0.027**	0.037***	0.018***
(s.e.)	(0.012)	(0.020)	(0.018)	(0.010)	(0.006)	(0.011)	(0.010)	(0.006)
Difference	0.093	−0.016	**0.242**	0.067	**−0.063***	−0.032	**−0.059**	**−0.037**
p-value	.18	0.90	0.02	0.27	0.00	0.34	0.04	0.03

Note. Control variables in all models: change in Gross State Product and change in state unemployment rate. Demographics and state level dummies are controlled for in the first stage prediction of earnings and income.
[a] The 1993 sample has 3065 recipients and 57440 non-recipients.
[b] The 1994 sample has 2774 recipients and 57434 non-recipients.
* = Significant at .10 level; ** = Significant at .05 level; *** = Significant at .01 level.

timate (if it were significant) would imply that earnings of an otherwise similar recipient living in a waiver state grew at 4.962 percent (.04962).

Table 1 also shows the value of the difference-in-difference approach in isolating the impact of the specific variable being examined. The difference-in-difference estimate is developed in the following way. The second coefficient in column 1 indicates that, in contrast to what would be a relatively lower growth in earnings for recipients in states with any work-related waivers, the earnings of a non-recipient grew 0.043 percentage points faster in a state with a work-related waiver compared with a non-recipient in a state without such a waiver.[6] While some of the difference between states in the earnings growth for non-recipients may be due to the fact that a few non-recipients are affected by waivers, much of it is likely due to unobservable factors that are correlated with the existence of a work-related waiver (e.g., changing attitudes toward work and welfare). The difference between the two estimates has been used to isolate the effect of the waiver from the unobservables that affect both recipients and non-recipients, resulting in the entry labeled "Difference," a difference-in-difference estimate. (Differences statistically significant at the .01 and .05 level are shown in boldface.) In this example the estimate is -0.081. A negative sign indicates that, were this to be a statistically significant estimate, the presence of any work-related waivers would in themselves have had a relatively negative impact on the growth of earnings among those who received public assistance. The p-value for statistical significance is shown under the difference-in-difference estimate. Here, the p-value of 0.23 indicates that the difference in the estimates is not significant, meaning that most of the observed state-level difference in recipients' earnings growth is due to unobservables rather than the work-related waivers themselves.

As the difference-in-difference estimates in Column 1 of Table 1 show, the variable combining all work-related waivers had no significant effect on earnings growth for this sample in any of the three time periods. This is consistent with the ambiguous theoretical predictions of the effects of both work requirement and work incentive waivers. However, the difference-in-difference estimate corresponding to this combination variable did have a negative and statistically significant effect on income growth in all three periods (column 5). For example, the difference-in-difference estimate for this variable in the 1993-94 time period (the second boldface entry in row 3) indicates that the family income of welfare recipients grew 0.068 percentage points more slowly than that of a non-recipient family living in the *same* state over that period. The negative effect is likely due to sanctions and other penalties for families who were unable to comply with the new rules. While it may be disturbing to find a negative effect, it should be noted that the magnitude is quite small. In sum, work-related waivers as a group are not associated with increased earnings growth on the part of welfare recipients in the full sample, but do appear to decrease the income growth of these families slightly.

The lack of effect of the combined work-related waivers on earnings growth could potentially be caused by a confounding of the influences of work requirement and work incentive waivers; when the effect of each of these is examined separately work-requirement waivers stand out for their negative effect. The work requirement waiver has a negative effect on earnings growth in all three time periods (column 2), though this estimate is statistically significant only for waivers implemented by the end of 1993 (the 1993-94 and 1993-95 results). The order of magnitude for the effects of 1993 work-requirement waivers, while still small, is much greater than the effects discussed earlier. The estimates imply that work requirement waivers caused family earnings of welfare recipients to grow approximately 0.25 percentage points more slowly than those of non-recipients in the same state.

There are three possible explanations for the negative effect of work requirements on the growth of earnings among those receiving welfare. First, this analysis estimates the change in *family* earnings growth. In families with more than one potential worker, one partner may choose to quit working if another is required to work. This is not likely to be the primary explanation, however, because most recipient families have only one potential worker. A second possibility is that some recipients may have worked at unreported jobs while receiving benefits. Edin and Lein (1997) report that this is relatively common. When a workfare type of waiver is implemented these recipients must report their work, and may no longer have time to work surreptitiously. This would result in an overall decrease in earnings.[7] The third explanation draws on the fact that many work requirement waivers allowed participation in a state-sponsored job training program in lieu of working. It may have been beneficial for some recipients who were originally working (whether reported or not) to participate in the job training program instead. The third explanation is consistent with the additional finding that the work requirement waiver had no significant effect on recipients' income growth (column 6). The only way income growth could remain constant while earnings growth falls would be if lower earnings growth was offset by increased growth in unearned income (including welfare benefits).

Turning to state work-incentive waivers also reveals an interesting pattern. As shown in column 3, the work incentive waivers did have a positive effect on earnings growth (but statistically significant only in the 1994-95 period). Simultaneously, work incentive waivers had a significant (but much smaller) negative effect on income growth (column 7). This pattern would be expected if the work incentive waivers helped recipients find paying jobs, but the increased wages triggered a large decrease in benefits. Although work incentive waivers were those that increased the earnings disregard (i.e., the wages a recipient could earn before experiencing a reduction in benefits), recipients still faced a steep phase-out period once their earnings exceeded the disregard.

Finally, it is possible to compare the effect of any type of waiver, whether work-related or not. These results are very similar to those of the variable that combines all work-related waivers. There is no significant impact on earnings growth (column 4) and a statistically significant, but quite small, negative effect on income growth (column 8). Again, sanctions and penalties are the logical explanation for this drop. Note that the measure of the income growth rate allows for recipients to leave the caseload during the period in question for all reasons, not just because of increased earnings. Ziliak, Figlio, Davis, and Connolly (2000) have analyzed the effect of waivers on caseload; the decrease in income growth could reflect the fact that many waivers were designed to reduce caseloads without necessarily increasing earnings.

Single Female Householders Only, Rural and Urban Residents Pooled

One weakness of the analysis shown in Table 1 is that it compares AFDC recipients with all non-recipients, which may not be the most appropriate control group. Table 2 presents the results of restricting the sample (of both recipients and non-recipients) to single female heads of household only. Everything else remains the same as before.

When columns 1 and 5 of Table 2 are compared with the full sample they show no differences in the pattern resulting from the variable that combines all work-related waivers, though the magnitudes are slightly different. As columns 4 and 8 indicate, there is also little difference in the pattern of the effect when all waivers are combined.[8]

There are some interesting differences in the effects of each type of work-related waiver when they are examined separately. When the sample is restricted to single female householders the effect of the work requirement variable on earnings growth, which in Table 1 was significant for 1993-94 and 1993-95 but not for the 1994-95 period, approaches significance ($p = .10$) for this period as well. The magnitude of the effect is also similar to that of the other two periods. The difference in this estimate compared with the corresponding estimate from the full sample is driven by the difference in the estimated effect on recipients. There is no difference in the effect for non-recipients (comparing row 8, column 2, of tables 1 and 2). However, these waivers had a negative ef-

TABLE 2. Differential Effect of Welfare Waivers on Growth in the Earnings and Income of Recipients of Public Aid, by Time Period (Single Female Householders Only)

Aid Recipient Status	Earnings: change in predicted growth of earnings with respect to kind of waiver				Income: change in predicted growth of income with respect to kind of waiver			
	Any work-related (1)	Work requirement (2)	Work Incentive (3)	Any waiver (4)	Any work-related (5)	Work requirement (6)	Work Incentive (7)	Any waiver (8)
				1993-1994				
Yes[a]								
coefficient	−0.009	−0.604***	0.285***	−0.022	−0.066***	−0.076**	−0.032	−0.043**
(s.e.)	(0.068)	(0.119)	(0.086)	(0.061)	(0.020)	(0.035)	(0.025)	(0.018)
No[a]								
coefficient	0.034	−0.364***	0.226***	−0.029	−0.009	−0.063**	0.024	−0.006
(s.e.)	(0.028)	(0.048)	(0.036)	(0.024)	(0.015)	(0.025)	(0.019)	(0.012)
Difference	−0.044	−0.240*	0.059	0.007	**−0.057****	−0.013	−0.056	−0.037*
p-value	0.56	0.06	0.53	0.92	0.02	0.76	0.93	0.09
				1993-1995				
Yes[a]								
coefficient	0.023	−0.419***	0.256***	−0.032	−0.068***	−0.021	−0.068***	−0.041**
(s.e.)	(0.072)	(0.126)	(0.092)	(0.064)	(0.018)	(0.032)	(0.024)	(0.016)
No[a]								
coefficient	0.055**	−0.110**	0.132***	−.065***	−0.013	−0.044*	0.001	−0.010
(s.e.)	(0.028)	(0.048)	(0.036)	(0.024)	(0.015)	(0.025)	(0.019)	(0.012)
Difference	−0.032	**−0.309****	0.124*	0.033	**−0.055****	0.023	−0.069	−0.031
p-value	0.67	0.02	0.09	0.63	0.02	0.57	0.64	0.14
				1994-1995				
Yes[b]								
coefficient	0.074	−0.081	0.281***	−0.024	−0.050**	−0.052	−0.034	−0.048***
(s.e.)	(0.071)	(0.128)	(0.104)	(0.062)	(0.020)	(0.037)	(0.030)	(0.018)
No[b]								
coefficient	0.010	0.142***	−0.018	−0.038*	0.007	0.003	−0.003	−0.004
(s.e.)	(0.026)	(0.043)	(0.038)	(0.022)	(0.014)	(0.024)	(0.021)	(0.012)
Difference	0.064	−0.223*	0.299	0.014	**−0.057****	−0.055	−0.031	**−0.044****
p-value	0.40	0.10	0.53	0.83	0.02	0.21	0.67	0.04

Note. Control variables in all models: change in Gross State Product and change in state unemployment rate. Demographics and state level dummies are controlled for in the first stage prediction of earnings and income.
[a] The 1993 sample has 2107 recipients and 16735 non-recipients.
[b] The 1994 sample has 1928 recipients and 16539 non-recipients.
* = Significant at .10 level; ** = Significant at .05 level; *** = Significant at .01 level.

fect on earnings growth for recipients in the restricted sample (−0.081, shown in row 7, column 2, of table 2), in contrast to the positive effect in the full sample (0.126, shown in row 7, column 2, of table 1). This potentially indicates that some effects of the later work requirement waivers on single female householders were obscured when the full sample was examined. However, the difference in the effect for recipients is not statistically significant (*p*-value = 0.24). As in the full sample, work requirement waivers had no significant effect on income growth for recipient families. Thus, the decrease in earnings growth is offset by growth in unearned income.

The work incentive variable shows two major changes in its effect. First, the positive effect on earnings growth in the 1994-95 period found in Table 1 (last row of column 3) is of about the same magnitude in the restricted sample, but in Table 2 is not statistically significant. Thus the apparent earnings benefit of the work incentive waivers disappears when the focus is only on families headed by single females. In part, this may be due to the smaller sample size used for the estimates in Table 2. However, it may suggest that the benefits accrue mainly to families with single male heads and/or two parents. The second difference in the effect of the work incentive waiver is that, though the effect on income growth remains negative (column 7), in the restricted sample it is not significant. It appears that families headed by single females were less likely to have earnings growth high enough to incur benefit reductions.

Full Sample, Rural and Urban Residents Separate

Labor market opportunities in rural areas often differ substantially from those in urban areas, so the analysis was repeated separately for rural and urban residents to see if welfare reform had the same impact in both areas. Like Tables 1 and 2, Tables 3 and 4 show estimates of differences in the earnings and income growth of welfare recipients and non-recipients for both the full sample and a sample restricted to single female householders. The estimates labeled "difference" in Tables 3 and 4 are difference-in-difference estimates that add the further condition of rural versus urban residence, but still correspond to the estimates labeled "difference" in Tables 1 and 2. For brevity, however, the coefficients for recipients and non-recipients have been omitted in Tables 3 and 4.

Table 3 shows the findings for the full sample. For urban residents, the effects of all types of waiver look very similar to that of the pooled sample. Of the significant variables, the only one with a positive effect is a work incentive waiver on earnings growth in the 1994-95 time period (and this is significant only if one is willing to accept a significance level of .10). This effect is somewhat smaller for the urban sample than the pooled sample. For all of the other significant variables, the effect is more negative in the urban sample than in the pooled sample. The differences in magnitudes of the effects for urban residents suggest that in

TABLE 3. Differential Effect of Welfare Waivers on Growth in the Earnings and Income of Recipients of Public Aid, by Time Period and Location of Residence (Full Sample, Initial Coefficients Omitted)

Location of Residence	Change in predicted earnings growth				Change in predicted income growth			
	Any work-related (1)	Work requirement (2)	Work Incentive (3)	Any waiver (4)	Any work-related (5)	Work requirement (6)	Work Incentive (7)	Any waiver (8)
				1993-1994				
Rural[a]								
Difference	−0.144	−0.255	−0.055	−0.085	−0.030	−0.065	−0.002	−0.024
p-value	0.33	0.26	0.79	0.52	0.44	0.25	0.97	0.48
Urban[b]								
Difference	−0.062	−0.262*	0.051	−0.028	**−0.074***	−0.017	**−0.070***	**−0.041***
p-value	0.42	0.06	0.60	0.68	0.00	0.61	0.00	0.01
				1993-1995				
Rural[a]								
Difference	−0.150	−0.257	−0.038	−0.049	−0.040	−0.086	0.006	−0.020
p-value	0.34	0.28	0.86	0.73	0.33	0.16	0.92	0.57
Urban[b]								
Difference	−0.087	−.305**	0.049	−0.039	**−0.079***	−0.025	**−0.075***	**−0.040**
p-value	0.28	0.04	0.63	0.59	0.00	0.50	0.00	0.03
				1994-1995				
Rural[c]								
Difference	0.222	0.042	0.389	−0.045	0.032	0.057	0.005	0.020
p-value	0.16	0.85	0.12	0.73	0.46	0.35	0.94	0.56
Urban[d]								
Difference	0.061	−0.061	0.217*	0.084	**−0.089***	−0.059	**−0.091***	**−0.055***
p-value	0.45	0.68	0.07	0.22	0.00	0.14	0.01	0.00

Note. Difference-in-difference estimates only shown here. Full results are available from the author upon request. Control variables in all models: change in Gross State Product and change in state unemployment rate. Demographics and state level dummies are controlled for in the first stage prediction of earnings and income.
[a]The 1993 full rural sample has 730 recipients and 14474 non-recipients.
[b]The 1993 full urban sample has 2335 recipients and 42966 non-recipients.
[c]The 1994 full rural sample has 591 recipients and 14009 non-recipients.
[d]The 1994 full urban sample has 2183 recipients and 43425 non-recipients.
* = Significant at .10 level; ** = Significant at .05 level; *** = Significant at .01 level.

general, waivers had a more negative (or less positive) effect on urban recipients than on all recipients as a group.

In contrast to the findings for urban residents, none of the difference-in-difference estimates is significant for any type of waiver for rural residents. Perhaps this is not surprising, since a large fraction of the pooled population consists of urban residents. However, rural residents comprise about 25 percent of the sample for both recipients and non-recipients, so the lack of significance for rural residents is not purely an artifact of small sample size. (There are 730 rural recipients in the 1993

TABLE 4. Differential Effect of Welfare Waivers on Growth in the Earnings and Income of Recipients of Public Aid, by Time Period and Location of Residence (Single Female Householders Only, Initial Coefficients Omitted)

Location of Residence	Change in predicted earnings growth				Change in predicted income growth			
	Any work-related (1)	Work require-ment (2)	Work Incentive (3)	Any waiver (4)	Any work-related (5)	Work require-ment (6)	Work Incentive (7)	Any waiver (8)
	1993-1994							
Rural[a]								
Difference	0.07	−0.060	0.005	0.127	0.034	−0.156*	0.103	0.036
p-value	0.69	0.81	0.99	0.39	0.54	0.07	0.65	0.46
Urban[b]								
Difference	−0.041	−0.308**	0.096	0.002	−0.071***	0.009	−0.076	−0.046*
p-value	0.62	0.04	0.14	0.98	0.01	0.86	0.41	0.06
	1993-1995							
Rural[a]								
Difference	0.027	0.041	−0.057	0.121	−0.011	−0.087	0.037	−0.012
p-value	0.89	0.88	0.51	0.47	0.85	0.30	0.79	0.82
Urban[b]								
Difference	−0.034	−.404***	0.160*	0.026	−0.066***	0.043	−0.089	−0.032
p-value	0.69	0.01	0.07	0.72	0.01	0.36	0.41	0.15
	1994-1995							
Rural[c]								
Difference	0.130	−0.214	0.419*	−0.102	−0.038	0.039	−0.077	−0.053
p-value	0.47	0.44	0.10	0.49	0.52	0.65	0.91	0.26
Urban[d]								
Difference	0.050	−0.225	0.275	0.038	−0.064**	−0.084*	−0.040	−0.043*
p-value	0.55	0.15	0.69	0.60	0.02	0.10	0.70	0.08

Note. Difference-in-difference estimates only shown here. Full results are available from the author upon request. Control variables in all models: change in Gross State Product and change in state unemployment rate. Demographics and state level dummies are controlled for in the first stage prediction of earnings and income.
[a]The 1993 sample has 450 recipients and 3868 non-recipients.
[b]The 1993 sample has 1657 recipients and 12867 non-recipients.
[c]The 1994 sample has 392 recipients and 3703 non-recipients.
[d]The 1994 sample has 1536 recipients and 12836 non-recipients.
* = Significant at .10 level; ** = Significant at .05 level; *** = Significant at .01 level.

sample and 591 in the 1994 sample.) Thus, it appears that the state-level welfare reform policies that had been implemented by the end of 1994 had no effect-good or bad-on the earnings or income growth of rural residents, but had a small detrimental effect on urban residents. There are several possible explanations for the differential effect on rural and urban residents. First, as Schiller (1999) notes, implementation of waivers often varied substantially across counties. Perhaps caseworkers in rural offices had more time to aid recipients in finding and keeping jobs, thereby insulating them from any negative effects. Second, it was noted earlier that the negative effect of work requirements on earnings growth may be due to recipients' participation in job training programs instead of work. Job training lowers earnings in the short run because participants are not working. If training was more readily available to urban residents, then the suppression of earnings would be smaller for rural residents. Third, any negative effect of work incentives on income growth is likely due to the steep phase-out of benefits when wages rise. If urban workers are more likely than their rural counterparts to earn higher wages, then the steep phase-out range is less likely to occur for rural recipients, leaving their incomes relatively constant.

Single Female Householders Only, Rural and Urban Residents Separate

Finally, distinct effects for rural and urban residence can be examined for the sample restricted to single female householders. As Table 4 indicates, the results for urban residents look even more like those of the pooled rural/urban sample than was the case when attention was not restricted.

The results differ slightly for rural residents. Two effects are significant for rural recipients. First is the effect of a work requirement waiver on income growth in 1993-94, which is negative and approaches significance at the .10 level. This estimate does not approach significance in any other sample. Thus, it appears that recipient families headed by single females and living in rural areas may have been somewhat more likely to incur sanctions or leave the welfare caseload as a result of work requirement waivers approved by the end of 1993. However, this effect does not appear to persist: The effect of a work requirement waiver on the income growth of this group is insignificant in the other two time periods.

The other effect that approaches significance for rural recipients is a positive impact of work incentive waivers on earnings growth in the 1994-95 period. A similar effect could also be seen in the unrestricted sample for urban residents alone and with urban and rural residents pooled. The effect is also similar in magnitude to the effect for rural residents in the unrestricted sample, but it is not significant in the latter case. The positive effect implies that work incentive waivers helped rural families headed by those single females who received welfare to earn additional income in the 1994-95 period.

DISCUSSION

Analyses of CPS data suggest that, overall, early welfare waivers containing work requirements had little impact on earnings growth and a negative, but small, impact on the income growth of recipients. The effects appear to have been somewhat more detrimental for urban recipients than for those living in rural areas. Most research on differences between urban and rural areas indicates that rural residents fare worse than their urban counterparts, so this result is somewhat surprising. It suggests that although rural residents in general may realize fewer economic gains, rural welfare recipients are somewhat insulated from the negative effects of welfare reform. Schiller (1999) argues that implementation varies widely across jurisdictions. He does not present evidence to suggest systematic variation across urban and rural jurisdictions, but it is possible that this does occur. If so, this could explain the lack of impact on rural recipients. Another explanation for the lack of impact of the work requirement waivers on the earnings growth of rural residents it that job training programs may not have been available so rural residents did not have the option of participating in these programs instead of working. Finally, the lack of effect of work incentives on income growth may be due to the fact that wages were lower in rural areas so rural recipients were less likely to incur losses in benefits as they began working at wage-earning jobs. The finding that waivers are less detrimental for rural residents is consistent with research by Davis, Connolly, and Weber (2001), who found that after controlling for differences in local economic conditions, being female or older has a smaller negative effect on the probability of finding a job for poor rural residents than for their urban counterparts.

POLICY IMPLICATIONS

Designers of welfare reform policies frequently argue that their policies will increase recipients' self-sufficiency. If so, then the policies should lead to higher earnings and income growth for former recipients. In this paper, two different samples from the Current Population Survey were used to estimate the effect of pre-PRWORA state level welfare waivers on the earnings and income growth of recipients compared with non-recipients over three time periods. Two variables combined waivers of various types: one combining work-related waivers only and another combining waivers of all types. Neither of these variables has any significant effect on earnings growth, regardless of the time period and sample used. Both waivers show a negative and (usually) statistically significant (but small) effect on income growth for a sample containing urban recipients only as well as one that pools urban and rural recipients. There is no significant effect of either variable on the income growth of rural recipients.

This study also separates the work-related waiver variable into two components: work requirements and work incentives. With two exceptions, the effect of the work requirement waiver on earnings growth is negative, though it is not always statistically significant. In the two cases in which it is positive, it is statistically insignificant. The negative effect may result from recipients who were previously working quitting their jobs in order to participate in job training programs or, for those who were working in violation of AFDC rules, in order to work at an approved job.

The work requirement waiver had an effect on income growth that closely approached significance (at the .10 level) in only two cases. Recipient families headed by single females living in rural areas of states with a work requirement saw lower income growth during the 1993-94 period than similar families in rural areas of states without such a waiver. Similarly, there was a negative impact on the income growth of urban recipient families headed by single females in the 1994-95 period. These negative effects are likely due to sanctions and families leaving the caseload.

The significance of work incentive waivers on earnings growth varies, but in cases where they are significant the effects are always positive. However, they have a significant (but small) negative effect on income growth in several instances.

While the results presented here cover only the effects of waivers approved by the end of 1993 and 1994, they are suggestive of the impacts that may have occurred in later years as well. Most of the later waivers, as well as PRWORA, have similar provisions as those studied here. The effects of these later reforms are now being examined directly using both the CPS and the newly released Survey of Program Dynamics.

Much of the discussion surrounding welfare reform has espoused the goal of "self-sufficiency" for recipients (though in practice, the stated purpose of much of the legislation was less lofty; the goal was to reduce the number of recipients). If former recipients are to attain self-sufficiency, then at minimum it will be necessary for family incomes to remain constant. Thus, it is crucial to understand what has happened economically to those who relied on welfare at the time of the new policies, whether or not they continued to receive benefits. This analysis suggests that those families are generally no better off, and are potentially worse off, as a result of welfare reform.

NOTES

1. The estimating equation is $\ln(\text{earn}_2) = X_2\beta_2 + e_2$, where $\ln(earn_2)$ is the natural log of earnings in Period 2, X_2 is a vector of demographic factors (listed in the text) and state dummy variables for families observed in Period 2, and e_2 is a residual from the censored normal distribution.

2. In this case, the predicted log earnings are simply equal to $X_1\beta_2$, *where* X_1 is the vector of demographics and state dummy variables for the Year 1 sample and β_2 is the vector of estimates obtained using the Year 2 sample.

3 The model is

$$(\widehat{LNEARN}_2 - LNEARN_1)_{is} = \alpha_0 + \alpha_1 \, WAIVER_s + \alpha_2 \, DGSP_s + \alpha_3 \, DUR_s + u_{is}$$

where i indexes individuals ($i = 1, \ldots , N$) and s indexes states, including the District of Columbia ($s = 1, \ldots ,51$). $\widehat{LNEARN}_2$ is predicted Period 2 log earnings, $LNEAR_1N$ is actual Period 1 log earnings, WAIVER is the welfare waiver variable, DGSP is the change in the state Gross State Product between Period 1 and Period 2, and DUR is the change in the state unemployment rate between Period 1 and Period 2. u_{is} is an error term that is assumed to be independent and normally distributed.

4. Work requirement waivers include those that change the Job Opportunity and Basic Skills Training Program (JOB) work exemption requirements, those that affect JOBS sanctions, and those that impose work requirements after some time limit is reached. Work incentive waivers are primarily those that increase the earnings disregard. Waivers that are not considered work related include a wide variety of provisions such as family caps (restricting benefit increases for women who bear additional children while on AFDC), adjustment to asset limits, and requirements that teenage mothers finish high school, among many others.

5. Schiller (1999) makes a compelling case that local discretion in county welfare offices can lead to wide variation in the degree to which particular provisions are implemented within a given state. This means that statewide waiver data may not provide accurate information about the ways in which welfare reforms actually affect recipients. Unfortunately, no data measuring implementation at the county level, especially in terms of the behavior of case workers, are available.

6. Not too much should be made of the point that this estimate is highly statistically significant, in contrast to the first estimate in column 1. The estimate for non-recipients is very precise because of the large sample size. Thus, all estimates for non-recipients are more likely to be statistically significant, even if they are small in magnitude.

7. Working recipients have an incentive to hide earnings from unreported jobs, so it is possible that earnings for this group of families are underreported in the CPS. If so, this would strengthen the argument: since fewer recipients are likely to be working in viola-

tion of AFDC rules after the work requirement is imposed, reported earnings in the second period are probably more accurate than first period earnings in waiver states. In this case, predicted earnings growth in waiver states would be overstated relative to that of non-waiver states. Thus, the actual effect of the waiver on earnings would be at least as large (in magnitude) as my estimates indicate.

8. While the signs of the 1993-94 and 1993-95 effect of the combined waiver variable on earnings growth differ between the full and restricted samples, these effects are not significant in either sample. The only consequential change is the lack of significance for the negative effect on income growth in the 1993-95 period for the restricted sample.

REFERENCES

Blank, R. M. (1997). *It Takes a Nation: A New Agenda for Fighting Poverty.* Princeton: Princeton University Press.

Brauner, S., & Loprest, P. (1999). *Where Are They Now? What States' Studies of People Who Left Welfare Tell Us* (The New Federalism: Issues and Options for States, Briefing paper A-32). Washington, DC: The Urban Institute.

Cancian, M. et al. (2001). *Work, Earnings, and Well-Being After Welfare: What Do We Know?* Paper presented at the conference on Welfare Reform and the Macro-Economy, November 19-20, 1999. Washington, DC: Joint Center for Poverty Research.

Connolly, L. S., & Segal, L. M. (2001). *Minimum Wage Legislation and the Working Poor.* Unpublished paper, University of Northern Colorado.

Crouse, G. (1999). *State Implementation of Major Changes to Welfare Policies, 1992-1998.* U.S. Department of Health and Human Services, Assistant Secretary for Planning and Evaluation, Office of Human Services Policy. <http://aspe.hhs.gov/hsp/Waiver-Policies99/policy_CEA.htm>.

Davis, E. E., Connolly, L. S., & Weber, B. A. (2001). *Employment Outcomes for Low-Income Adults in Rural and Urban Labor Markets.* Unpublished paper, University of Minnesota.

Deavers, K. L., & Hoppe, Robert A. (1992). Overview of the Rural Poor in the 1980s. In C. M. Duncan (ed.), *Rural Poverty in America,* 3-20. Westport, CT: Auburn House.

Edin, K., & Lein, L. (1997). *Making Ends Meet: How Single Mothers Survive Welfare and Low-Wage Work.* New York: Russell Sage Foundation.

Ehrenberg, R. G., & Smith, R. S. (1994). *Modern Labor Economics: Theory and Public Policy,* 5. New York: HarperCollins.

Findeis, J. et al. (1992). *Poverty and Work: Utilization of Resources Among the Rural Poor.* Final Report, Ford Foundation Rural Poverty Program and Rural Economic Policy Program of the Aspen Institute.

Findeis, J., & Jensen, L. (1998). Employment Opportunities in Rural Areas: Implications for Poverty in a Changing Policy Environment. *American Journal of Agricultural Economics,* 80(5), 1000-07.

Moffitt, R. A., & Gottschalk, P. (1995). *Trends in the Autocovariance Structure of Earnings in the U.S.: 1969-1987* (Working Papers in Economics, 355). Baltimore: The Johns Hopkins University, Department of Economics.

Moffitt, R. A. (1996). The Effect of Employment and Training Programs on Entry and Exit from the Welfare Caseload. *Journal of Policy Analysis and Management, 15*(1, Winter), 32-50.

Moffitt, R. A. (1999). *The Effect of Pre-PRWORA Waivers on AFDC Caseloads and Female Earnings, Income, and Labor Force Behavior.* Working Paper, Joint Center on Poverty Research.

Schiller, B. R. (1999). State Welfare-Reform Impacts: Content and Enforcement Effects. *Contemporary Economic Policy, 17*(2, April), 210-22.

Tapogna, J., & Witt, T. (1998). *Making the Transition to Self-Sufficiency in Oregon* (Report prepared for the Oregon Coalition of Community Non-Profits Under Subcontract to Children First for Oregon). Portland, OR: ECONorthwest.

U.S. Council of Economic Advisers (1997). *Explaining the Decline in Welfare Receipt, 1993-1996.* Technical Report.

Weber, B. A., Acock, A. C., & Goetz, K. W. (1991). *Defining Rural: Implications of Alternative Definitions for Oregon Rural Policy* (Legislative Discussion Paper). University of Oregon: Rural Policy Research Group.

Ziliak, J. P., Figlio, D. N., Davis, E. E., & Connolly, L. S. (2000). The Decline in AFDC Caseloads: Welfare Reform or the Economy? *Journal of Human Resources, 35*(3, Summer), 570-586.

Ziliak, J. P., Figlio, D. N., Davis, E. E., & Connolly, L. S. (1997). *Accounting for the Decline in AFDC Caseloads: Welfare Reform or Economic Growth?* (Institute for Research on Poverty Discussion Paper 1151-97). Madison: University of Wisconsin.

Index

Acock, A. C., 157
Acs, G., 130
Ahluwalia, S., 68,78,84,85,86
Ali, E., 42,47
Allison, P., 54
Altman, B. E., 15
Anderson, J. R., 107
Anderson, N. J., 67
Andes, S., 2,4
Aneshensel, C. S., 48
Annie E. Casey Foundation, 42
At-risk populations, 120-121

Bandura, A., 98,121,125
Barnard, K., 50
Barriers, to employment, 14,67-68
    educational, 17
    personal, 17-18
Bassuk, S., 98,103,108
Becker, G. S., 43
Betz, N. E., 121
Birkimer, J. C., 50
Blank, R. M., 155
Blome, J., 67,87
Bogen, K., 130
Bourdieu, P., 43
Boyd, J. M., 49,50
Brauner, S., 152
Brooks, M., 44,45,59,67,96,98,103,
    108,115
Brumley, H. E., 67,68
Buckner, J., 44,45,59,67,96,98,103,115
Budig, M., 44
Burke, V., 2
Burr, B., 45
Burtless, G., 42
Burton, B., 130

Callahan, S., 130
Cancian, M., 153
Career search efficacy, 121,126-127. *See
    also* Self-efficacy
Career Search Efficacy Scale (CSES),
    121-122
Carlson, V., 47
Casten, R., 98,116
Cave, G., 67
Center for Epidemiological Studies
    Depression Scale (CES-D),
    50-51
Cervantes, P., 50
Chapin Hall Center for Children, 130
Chartrand, J. M., 120
Chavkin, W., 130
Cherlin, A., 130
Child care, 47
    as facilitator to employment, 18-19
    Illinois Job Advantage Program and,
        23
Child outcomes
    maternal depression and literacy as
        predictors of, 75-78
    parenting behavior, 78-79
Child Support Enforcement program, 4
Cho, Y, I., 48
Clark, V. A., 48
Coiro, M. J., 70
Coll, C. G., 97,101
Community Kitchens program, research
    study of, 122-126,127
Connolly, L. S., 3,130,152,154,157,
    165,171
Control, personal sense of, 35
Corcoran, M., 14
Crittenden, K. S., 2,4
Crouse, G., 154,161

Sawhill, I., 130
Schiller, B. R., 169,171
Schwartz, D., 16,35
Schwarzer, R., 98,102,105,106,112
Seecombe, K., 96,97
Seefeldt, K., 14,67
Self-efficacy, 3,98-99,110-111,
    114,121. *See also* Career
    search efficacy
  welfare-to-work programs and,
    125-126
Seltzner, S. P., 15
Shanahan, M. J., 67
Shaw, L., 45
Sholomskas, D., 50
Siefert, K., 14
Sigmon, S. T., 108
Smith, R. S., 154
Smith, Rojas, 3,4
Snow, C., 72
Social ecological model, 15,38
Solberg, V. S., 121,122,123,127
Solomon-Fears, C., 2
Spalter-Roth, R., 45
Spar, K., 2
Sterrett, E. A., 98,122
Strong, D., 88
Substance abuse
  Illinois Job Advantage Program
    and, 23-24
  state programs for monitoring,
    140
Surrey, L. A., 97,101
Swinton, D. H., 120
Syner, C. R., 107
Synthetic panels, 157-158
  construction of, 158-159

Tapogna, J., 155
Taylor, R., 98,116
Telleen, Sharon, 2,4,15
Temporary Assistance to Needy
    Families (TANF), 1,8,9,
    14,66,130

and impact on minority families, 97-98
  goal of, 96-97
  Illinois program of, 46-47
Theodore, N., 47
Thoits, P. A., 48
Thompson, D., 50
Tobit estimation, 157-158
Tolman, R., 14
Transportation, 47
Trickett, E. J., 15,26

U. S. Council of Economic Advisers,
    154
U. S. Department of Health and Human
    Services, 46

Vernon, S. W., 50

Waite, L. J., 44
Waivers, 154-156
  effects of, on earnings and income,
    161-170
  income and, 171-173
  research study on effects of, 156-161
Walters, K. B., 96,97
Weaver, K., 130
Weber, B. A., 157,171
Weil, 8
Weinfield, N. S., 72
Weingarten, A., 97,101
Weissman, M. M., 50
Welfare reform
  identifying effects of, 159-160
  measures of, 160-161
Welfare waivers. *See* Waivers
Welfare, trends in, 51-53
Welfare-to-work programs
  self-efficacy and, 125-126
  studies of, 15
Well-being, trends in, 53
  research findings of, 56-57

Williams, K. B., 98,110,111
Winn, E., 130
Wise, P. H., 130
Witt, T., 175
Wolfe, B., 67,110,111
Wolfe, S. L., 98
Women's health
　research study of state programs
　　　monitoring, 132-145
　welfare reform and, 130
Woodcock, R. W., 72
Work history, as facilitator to
　　employment, 18
Work incentives waivers, 155
Work Pays program, 46

Work requirements, 152
　waivers, 154-156
Work, trends in, 51-53
Working conditions, as facilitator to
　　employment, 18

Yoshinobu, L., 108

Zaslow, M. J., 67,68,69,70,78,84,85,
　　86,87
Ziliak, J. P., 152,154,165
Zima, N., 123
Zuroff, D. C., 50